To: Debra

Health
Is
WEALTH

Thank you for getting
on the health train!
Love you!

Dr. Janine Jazzy Jordan

Health
Is
WEALTH

How to Live Without Cancer, High Blood Pressure,
Diabetes, Obesity, and Heart Disease,
Where You Feel Good All the Time
and Have Plenty of Energy

James "Jazzy" Jordan

This book is not intended to be a substitute for the medical advice of a licensed physician. The reader should consult with their doctor in any matters relating to his/her health.

CONTENTS

PROLOGUE

My name is James "Jazzy" Jordan, and I believe that a plant-based diet is the only way to decrease your chances of getting cancer, high blood pressure, diabetes, and heart problems. So, why would you not choose to save your life? That should be the most important thing to us. I have eaten a plant-based diet for the last 27 years, and I have enjoyed every minute of it. It is never too late to change your life; as long as you are breathing, you have time. I have gone on all sorts of journeys over the last 27 years, looking for the best way to eat. I have listened to all the professionals, eaten only raw food, and completed a 21-day water-only fast. I have done all of this to learn what's best for our bodies and, hopefully, I can help with your journey. If you consider this path, let me save you some steps and help you get to the promised land.

My book, *Health Is Wealth*, is dedicated to everyone looking to live a healthy life. If you feel that you are losing the battle for your health, you probably are. However, we can change that. If you do not consume the proper food, you will lose the battle more quickly. It has been said that we take another step closer to the grave every day. What I am looking to do is make it a longer walk. Today, no matter where you are living, you are very likely breathing polluted air and eating poisonous food. Our civilization has encouraged us, through advertising and education, to adopt many practices that make the human body sick, ugly, tired, and loaded with disease.

Supermarkets carry more than 7,000 items processed from whole foods; these are non-foods. The wholesome nutrition has been removed and replaced with synthetic poisonous chemicals. Fast food outlets, restaurants, animal protein, and supermarkets have helped create the sickest nation on the planet. Do you realize that more than 70 percent of Americans, including 30 percent of youth under 17, are suffering from chronic diseases and disorders?[1] These are the medicated incurables. Everyone else, with the exception of those who are using a simple vegetarian or vegan diet, self-medicate with laxatives, aspirin, sleeping pills, tranquilizers, and alcohol. Life is too short for us to live without having the benefits of health.

If you are sick, tired, and sluggish, it is because you do not understand what proper nutrition is, so you put anything in your mouth. The first thing we do in the morning after fighting to get up from a sleep-deprived night is grab a cup of coffee. We must have coffee; we cannot function without it. Why is that?

Since we are depriving our bodies of the proper nutrition that is needed to function the way it is designed to, we must have a stimulant to get through the day. The minute we are up, we turn to coffee. After crude oil, coffee is the most sought-after commodity in the world, putting it ahead of commodities like natural gas, gold, oil, sugar, and corn. The coffee industry is worth over $100 billion worldwide. Globally, we drink over 500 billion cups of coffee every year; of that, 14 billion are Italian espressos. Fifty percent of Americans drink coffee every day. The average person drinks three and a half cups of coffee every day, and if we are not drinking coffee, we are grabbing an energy drink.[2]

Now you have had a cup or two of coffee you can get through the morning, but at lunch, you need another stimulant to get you through the

[1]	Center for Disease Control and Prevention CDC 24/7: Saving Lives, Protecting People www.cdc.gov/cdctv/emergencypreparednessandresponse/cdc-24-7.html

[2]	Global Coffee Industry Facts & Statistics of 2014-2015 May 29, 2015 | 10:09 am Wevio www.wevio.com › Blog › Global Coffee Industry Facts & Statistics of 2014-2015

remainder of the day. Sales of energy drinks and shots will grow to a value of $21.5 billion by 2017.[3]

We have fallen into the trap of not taking care of ourselves and depending on a stimulant to get us through the day. If we do not have our coffee, most of us are cranky and not very lovable. Without an energy drink in the afternoon, our work production falls drastically because we can barely keep our eyes open, and that is after getting eight hours of sleep. Our bodies are telling us that we are not taking care of them, but we tend to ignore them and keep turning to a stimulant. After a day of stimulants, we need a downer, so we go for alcohol or a tranquilizer to get to sleep.

What is the solution? The solution is changing your habits, starting with a better diet. By changing to a healthy diet (of course, I suggest it's plant-based), you will not need energy drinks or coffee or anything else to get you through the day; your body will be vibrant and alive. Please do not do what I did by falling into the trap of calling yourself a vegetarian and still eating junk.

I switched from a standard American diet to being a vegetarian, and for many years, I was an unhealthy vegetarian: someone who eats the crap that has flooded the market and is called health food. Remember this, if it is processed, manmade, founded in the frozen food department and you cannot pronounce the names of the ingredients it is more than likely unhealthy.

We do not need processed foods loaded with sodium and sugar in our diet. Food manufacturers care about money, not our health. They are brilliantly skilled at manufacturing goods that sound great but are not good for us. If we want vegetarian or vegan, they will give us vegetarian or vegan, but it may kill us in the process.

Without eating animal flesh, we can still develop high blood pressure, diabetes, and clogged arteries and become overweight. We can feel good

---

[3]   Energy Drinks and Shots: U.S. Market Trend Jan 29, 2013 137 Pages - Pub ID: LA4873762 www.packagedfacts.com/Energy-Drinks-Shots

about ourselves being vegetarian or vegan, but if our diet is not nutritious, it does not matter.

If you are going to go plant-based, you should go all the way, and that is vegan. There are no shortcuts when it comes to your health.

Research shows that pollution of the bloodstream from mindless eating affects our health more than the air we breathe. The emphasis I am placing in this book will be on a low-starch, low-protein, low-fat, plant-based vegan diet. Sprouts or greens are high in enzymes, vitamins, and alkaline materials that will provide all the nutrients necessary for the body.

What I did was change my way of life, not my diet. My food became low starch, low protein, and low fat. I got rid of all the processed foods I was eating, and in 21 days, I got my blood pressure down from 180/100 to 120/70 and dropped 20 pounds—just by making a few simple changes in my life. If you are eating processed foods from the health food section, and that is not good for you, just imagine what most people are eating every day and how bad that is for them. We will not have to worry so much about health care if we change the way we eat.

It is amazing how much we know about our cars and how little we are aware of our bodies. We know what type of gas to use and the type and size of the tires that go on our cars, and we have warning signs to tell us when we are running out of gas or when to change the oil. But, what do you know about your body? Believe it or not, our bodies give us warning signs. When you wake up with a headache, that is a warning sign that something is wrong. When you do not have a bowel movement for two or three days, that is a warning sign; that is not healthy, no matter what anyone tells you. We should have a bowel movement every day. If your dog or cat did not relieve itself every day, you would become concerned. So, what about you?

If you answer yes to any of these questions, you should read on:

- Do you suffer from high blood pressure?
- Do you have diabetes?
- Do you know anyone with cancer?
- Do you want to live a healthy life?
- Do you have erectile dysfunction?
- Do you love yourself and your family?

I know I can help you restart your life in 21 days. I will show you how you should eat, what to eat, give you recipes that will make your life healthier and happier. You will not only be pleased with yourself, but your significant other will be thrilled.

CHAPTER ONE

Put Down the Chicken and Back Away

In the summer of 1990, I was working in New York City, living on top of the world, when I met the woman who would change my life. She was visiting my boss, Rick. Rick's office was the corner office, located two doors down from mine, and she had to pass by me in order to get to Rick.

I was at my desk, working on the computer, when I felt a cool summer breeze as she moved past me. I looked up just in time to see this lovely angel floating by. I was like Jack Nicholson playing the Joker in the 1989 Batman movie when he first saw Kim Basinger as Vicki Vale: the only thing he could say was "stop the press." I felt the same way. I dropped everything I was doing and went to Rick's office and asked Betty, his executive assistant, "Who was that?" She told me her name was Linda and that she was a professor at NYU. I asked Betty to ask Linda to stop by my office on her way out.

When she had finished her business with Rick, Betty delivered my message. When Linda arrived, I introduced myself and invited her out to lunch. She agreed, and lunch was set for the next week. Not knowing much about her, I picked a German restaurant. Although I do not like German food, it was close to the office. I had no idea that she was a vegetarian, so my choice of restaurants was not the best. Fortunately, she was not uptight. We had a great time, even though we were not into German food. We talked about what it was like to be a vegetarian. I had not thought much about becoming a vegetarian or vegan.

She already had a boyfriend, so my luck was out, but after lunch we became instant friends. We would have lunch from time to time, and I got introduced to a vegetarian lifestyle. I am so thankful to Linda for the introduction.

Four months after meeting Linda, on October 22, 1990, I decided to become a vegetarian. I was working all kind of crazy hours and eating very poorly—fried food, steak, junk food late at night—and it was making me feel sick and tired. I was waking up tired after getting eight hours of sleep, like I had just gone to bed. I had constant headaches and was feeling very sluggish.

So, I decided to try Linda's way of life because she was healthy and energetic. At first, I stopped eating animal flesh and drinking alcohol to see how that would make me feel. I immediately felt better and more in control of what I was doing. I had a very demanding job at Polygram Label Group, a music company. My job was to market artists like Salt-N-Pepa and P.M. Dawn, and many others. It was not an easy transition for me because I was around nothing but carnivores and borderline alcoholics. Everywhere we went, there were three things: alcohol, bad food, and a great time.

I also worked with the fabulous E 40. He called and wanted to meet about his new release, so I flew to see him at his office in Vallejo, California. In the middle of the meeting, it was just the two of us, he abruptly stopped and said, "Wait a minute, I need to ask you a question." E 40 looked me in the eyes and asked, "Is it true that you do not eat meat?"

I said, "That's right."

He said, "Help me understand. So that means no chicken, fish, or steak?"

I said, "Yes."

He then asked, "Are you allergic to it?"

I said, "No, personal choice."

He started shaking his head in disbelief. You, see 40 stands about 6' 3" tall and weighs around 300 pounds, so for him to be around someone that did not consume meat did not make any sense to him. He could not wrap his head around why someone would decide to do that.

I think I was the first vegetarian he had ever met in his life. I explained it to him. I said, "40, think about it like this: for every piece of chicken or steak I do not have, there's more for you."

He looked puzzled for a second, and then he said, "Yeah, my man" and gave me a fist bump.

Why vegan when you could be vegetarian, or keep eating animal flesh and dairy? There are so many answers to that question, and the best one I have is that you love yourself, your mate, and your family and want to live a healthy life.

I have learned that a plant-based diet can save your life. We do not have to suffer from strokes or heart attacks. High blood pressure can be regulated and diabetes can be controlled (and sometimes eliminated), all by changing your diet. I was fortunate because I was in pretty good shape, and it was easy to change my diet, but I know that it is not easy for everyone.

A meat eater loves the taste of animal flesh. We eat animals because of habit, convenience, tradition, and taste. However, with willpower, you can make a change. If you need help, I will be your coach, your guide, the one who helps you walk past the junk food and put down the shakes and fries.

For those of you who are happy with a big plate of guts or liver on your plate, have you ever stopped to think about what the functions of the liver and intestines are? Just in case you have forgotten, the liver's job is to filter all impurities out of the body, and the intestines . . . enough said. Most people are aware of the functions of these organs and will still fry them, sit down with a bottle of hot sauce, and feast on chicken gizzards, livers, or chitterlings. Sometimes I wonder: Do most people ever stop to think about what they are dropping in their pie holes? I do not believe they do.

Intestines are consumed all over the world. Korean cuisine offers *makchang gui*, a form of grilled pork intestines, while French cuisine has *tri canailles*, also grilled, and China has *jiangsu chaos dachang*, in which the intestines are stir-fried. Many countries around the world consume sheep or cow intestines.

If you feed yourself dead or poisonous food, then it's only going to kill you sooner. There's no question that we are all going to die; the question is what your quality of life will be like while you are living.

Man's basic physiology has not changed in millions of years. He still has the digestive tract of a fruitarian animal (gorilla). There is no significant digestive similarity between man and meat-eating animals. I believe that man has made an evolutionary error by introducing animal products and cooked food into his diet.

Meat and eggs are not healthy foods. They are high in cholesterol. When excessively heated, medicated animal products causes toxic waste products of protein metabolism that will rot in the intestine, leading to degenerative diseases such as heart disorders, cancer, leukemia, and gout.

Dairy products are mucus inducing, loaded with chemicals, and difficult to digest once pasteurized and combined with other foods. Many people are allergic to dairy. Dairy food is one of the leading causes of colds, respiratory disorders, and artery degeneration.

Milk is central to our development; it is universally accepted and understood that a mother's milk is unequivocally what nature has planned for the growth of babies across all species. Not only does it provide essential nourishment, but by drinking it, a baby also shares its mother's immune system and gets the right balance of fats, proteins, vitamins, hormones, and enzymes for development.

After a mother has finished nursing her baby, something odd happens—a cow takes over! This makes us the only mammal on Earth that is never really weaned off milk. No species on the planet except humans consumes milk in adulthood or, as a matter of fact, consumes the milk of another species!

In fact, most people believe that their health will be jeopardized if they do not consume dairy products. Cow milk is often described as nature's most wholesome food. Our "nutritional education" in schools (funded in part by the dairy industry) teaches us that dairy products form one of the main food groups we all need for proper nutrition, and with the most powerful congressional leaders in Washington receiving campaign contributions from the National Dairy Council, we can be assured that dairy products will continue to be advertised as food that is "necessary" for good health. The bottom line is that cow's milk is meant for calves to grow and not for humans. We are not meant to be drinking cow's milk, at least not in the quantities that we do, especially into adulthood.

My own research, and research publications (many being medical journals), clearly shows that eating a plant-based diet has significant protective values in a toxic environment. It can regenerate a sick body into a healthy one, and you can maintain life in excellent health.

Here is a challenge for you. For 21 days, give up all animal products and replace those with raw and cooked vegan dishes. Pay close attention to how you feel after the 21 days, and then prepare yourself a meal typical of what you usually ate. Devastating effects will be quickly evident after you are back to your regular diet. You will experience a lack of energy, heaviness of the body, and a mental stupor, unless you drink coffee or energy drinks after your meal.

After 21 days of abstinence from dairy products, such as milk, yogurt, and cheese, all of the symptoms of a cold will more than likely be induced. This is the body's way of cleaning itself, and these undesirable effects are more convincing than all of the arguments for veganism. You have a choice. You can be a lifeless food addict with inferior health, or you can become a vegan and experience the joy of living.

I guarantee you once your body adapts to a plant-based diet, you will not enjoy what you previously dined on.

10 Reasons to Go Vegan

1. Stop harming animals

2. If you are healthy, you will be happier

3. Vegan and raw foods are delicious

4. Good health for a lifetime

5. If we stop feeding for slaughter, no one on the planet needs to be hungry

6. Lose weight and have more energy

7. Save the planet

8. It's time for a change

9. Look sexy and be sexy; sexy is feeling good

10. By adopting a vegan diet, you can personally save up to 95 animals a year, and thousands during your lifetime.

The protein argument

You may believe that the only way to get protein in your diet is by eating meat. Fortunately, that is false; there are many ways to get enough protein without touching a piece of chicken or a hamburger. Harming animals is not necessary to get our protein. We kill 60 billion land animals yearly—more than 30 million daily.

I love this quote from William Ralph Inge:

> "We have enslaved the rest of the animal creation, and have treated our distant cousins in fur and feathers so badly that beyond doubt if they were able to formulate a religion, they would depict the Devil in human form."
>
> – **William Ralph Inge**[4]

Almost all foods, with the exception of fats and fruits, contain some protein. Beans, peas, nuts, seeds, vegetables, grains, and soy products are exceptionally high in protein.

It is believed that protein is an essential part of our diet because it provides energy, helps us grow, and allows our body to heal cuts and make other "repairs."

Dr. T. Colin Campbell, author of *The China Study*, has a lot to say about cancer and protein. Dr. Colin Campbell, who grew up on a dairy farm, has researched the need for protein for more than 50 years, concluding that too much protein can lead to cancer and a very unhealthy diet.

Take a look at the comparison chart on my website:

www.jamesjazzyjordan.com

---

[4] William Ralph Inge Quotes - BrainyQuote. (n.d.). Retrieved from http://www.brainyquote.com/quotes/quotes/w/williamral104044.ht

CHAPTER TWO

No Contest—We Win: We Are the Sickest Nation on the Planet

We are seeing more overweight people all over the country: in big cities, small cities, and country towns. We are putting on so much weight, and there is an undeniable reason for it: our food choices. We need to learn how to eat again and what to eat. We are consuming more and more food; a single Whopper® is not big enough; we now need double patties. All of our food choices are bigger—not better, just bigger.

Most of the food you buy at stores these days is loaded with sugar and sodium. One-third of deaths in the United States are caused by heart diseases, strokes, and other heart-related diseases. Also, heart diseases and strokes are the leading causes of death worldwide. In 2013, according to a report by the American Heart Association (AHA), cardiovascular diseases killed 801,000 Americans. These are deaths from strokes and heart-related conditions, which include heart attacks, heart failures, as well as valve and artery diseases. Coronary heart disease alone caused 370,000 deaths in the United States that year, according to the AHA.

About 795,000 people in the United States had a stroke in 2013. These strokes caused nearly 129,000 deaths. Approximately 750,000 Americans had a heart attack in 2013. Those heart attacks resulted in 116,000 deaths in 2013, the researchers reported.

The report also noted significant racial differences. The risk of a stroke in blacks is nearly twice as likely than that of whites, according to the report. The research found that almost half of all black people have some form of heart or stroke-related disease, because of diet.

Again, the AHA reported that, between 2003 and 2004 and between 2011 and 2012, the proportion of Americans eating a healthy diet rose from 0.2 percent to 0.6 percent among children and from 0.7 percent to 1.5 percent among adults. Even so, nearly 160 million Americans were overweight or obese (69 percent of adults and 32 percent of children) in 2009–2012.[5]

During that time, about 17 percent of adults (13 million) were obese, according to the AHA's 2016 Heart Disease and Stroke Statistics Update.

From 2009 to 2012, almost half of Americans had total cholesterol of 200 mg/dL or higher. And one-third (80 million) of Americans had high blood pressure, the report said. Nine percent of Americans have been diagnosed with diabetes, and 35 percent have pre-diabetes, the AHA noted. If we all start eating healthily, these numbers will decline very quickly.

I believe people would do better if they knew better. We cannot keep doing the same thing and hope for different results. That's why I am here, to show you another way. We have to get off the couch, put down the remote and do some exercise, start growing our food again, and learn to make better food choices. It's all about how we put our food together and what we choose to put in our mouths.

Let's talk about proper digestion. Most people suffer from digestive disorders. Many are treated for their disorders, and others experience

---

[5] "Heart Disease Now Kills 1 of Every 3 Americans - WebMD." hatp://wwwmd.com/ heart-disease/news/20151216/

symptoms of indigestion, lack of vigor, headaches, dizziness, insomnia or a need for many hours of sleep, not knowing the cause.

Indigestion stems from anxiety, eating highly processed food, eating hurriedly, reduced concentration of digestive juices, eating excessively, and not chewing food thoroughly. The biggest villain is serving two concentrated foods that are hard to digest at the same meal.

The human digestive tract was not made to be a receptacle for an eight-course meal containing a wide variety of foods. As long as the body's vitality is high, you can lead the life of a gourmet. In time, bouts of indigestion become more frequent.

The typical combination of meat, potatoes, butter or margarine, a glass of milk, along with various highly processed carbohydrates (bread, pasta) has produced the sickest nation on the planet.

Proteins require acidic digestive juices, while starch and sweet food require alkaline. We cannot digest both at the same time. Dairy products are highly alkaline, so they interfere with meat digestion. Fat interferes with protein digestion.

Poorly combined foods remain in the digestive tract for hours. In this warm environment, it rots or ferments, producing a vast range of poisons, headaches, and an unloving temperament.

Vegetables take longer to digest than fruit, and combining them in a single meal can cause fermentation. If we listen to our bodies, we will discover which food combinations are best for healthy digestion and vitality.

According to the Academy of Nutrition and Dietetics, an evidence-based review[6] showed that a vegan diet was associated with a lower risk of death from ischemic heart disease. Vegans appear to have lower low-density lipoprotein cholesterol levels, lower blood pressure, and lower

---

[6] Eating more plant protein associated with lower risk of ... (n.d.). Retrieved from http://www.kurzweilai.net/eating-more-plant-protein-associated-with-lower-risk-o

rates of hypertension and type 2 diabetes than meat-eaters. Vegans also tend to have lower body mass index, lower overall cancer rates, and a lower risk of chronic disease.

CHAPTER THREE

HOW TO EAT TO
LIVE OR DIE

Organic live food is our best Medicare, a ticket to prolonging our lives. Eat those natural foods that appeal to you most. Advance your diet according to the dictates of your body and the type of work you do. Only the subconscious knows our authentic needs. Forget charts, tables, and nutritionists; they are only for civilized food addicts. Do not use your teeth to crush hard food. If it's hard to masticate, it is forbidden.

Natural foods are in their most nutritious state when eaten uncooked, picked right from the orchard or garden. Cooking destroys most of the enzymes, lecithin, many vitamins, and much of the protein. As much as 85 percent of the original nutrition may be lost by cooking our food.

On a raw food diet, we get higher nutritional value from our food; hence, you eat less. Considering the overpopulation and overweight problems we have and that so many people are starving, it is a crime against humanity to waste food and raise so many animals for slaughter. The cost of feeding animals to serve us is out of control. Here is what Professor David Pimentel has to say:

"If all the grain currently fed to livestock in the United States were consumed directly by people, the number of people who could be fed would be nearly 800 million or, if those grains were exported, it would boost the U.S. trade balance by $80 billion a year."[7]

The body cannot heal or clean itself when it is working overtime digesting animal flesh and processed food. Our digestive systems are comprised of a group of organs working together to convert food into energy and the basic nutrients to feed the entire body. Food passes through a long tube inside the body known as the alimentary canal or the gastrointestinal (GI) tract. The alimentary canal is made up of the oral cavity, pharynx, esophagus, stomach, small intestine, and large intestine. In addition to the alimentary canal, there are several important accessory organs that help our body digest food. So, if we put live food (plants) in our body, it will be consumed quickly and turn into energy.

When we feed ourselves dead food (meat), it will take longer to digest, and we will get very little energy from it. That's why, after a big meal of something like a steak dinner, we are often tired and only want to sleep. If we are not taking in the right food, our body will see it as an enemy and will try to get it out of us as quickly as possible, making it difficult to work on anything other than digestion. To be healthy we must eat live food.

---

[7] Livestock Grain Could Feed 800 Million | EurekAlert ... (n.d.). Retrieved from http://www.eurekalert.org/pub_releases/1997-08/CUNS-LGCF-110897.php

CHAPTER FOUR

HOLD UP, WAIT A MINUTE— NO MORE FRIED FOOD!

Do you want to know why this is the sick and tired generation?

Currently, Americans get 60 percent of their daily total fat from added fats and oils, a large portion of which comes from fried foods. Take the latest national surveys on weight. More than 70 percent of all Americans are considered overweight or obese (meaning they have a body mass index greater than 25), according to the Centers for Disease Control and Prevention.

Multiple studies have pointed to oil consumption, particularly saturated fat, as one of the key dietary contributors to chronic diseases including heart disease, cancer, diabetes, and hypertension. It is not surprising that it is recommended that we cut out fried foods from our diets, but here are some more reasons to do so: pesticides are frequently found in the oil used in fried foods, and the oil is depleted of minerals and vitamins. Foods fried in this oil will simply attack our body's ability to fight diseases, thereby weakening our immunity to diseases in the long run. Most fried foods contain MSG (Monosodium glutamate), a toxic salt that's added to enhance the taste of "dead food," and it is full of fat. And fat is high in calories.

Consuming too many calories leads to being overweight, which leads to problems such as diabetes and heart disease. A Spanish study found that people who ate the most calories in fried food were most likely to become obese. The nutritional value of fried food is poor. Fried proteins are converted into acrolein, a known carcinogen. Heating vegetable oil above 300 degrees Fahrenheit damages the oil, causing toxin formation in the fried foods.

Fried foods clog arteries and lead to strokes. Studies have shown that eating fried foods can be a contributor to Alzheimer's. Fried foods lead to inflammation, which leads to joint problems. Modified, processed, and fried foods do not break down in the body properly, remaining in kidneys, liver, intestines, prostate, and colon for extended periods of time as toxins. Fried food breading soaks up nearly every drop of the oil, so eating fried chicken and pan pizza is like drinking oil straight from the vat. Eating fried foods will increase our low-density or "bad" cholesterol.

In restaurants, typically, hydrogenated or partially hydrogenated oils are used—which are other words for trans fat. Trans fat is a manmade fat that improves the shelf life of processed foods, but at the same time, raises our cholesterol and increases the risk of heart diseases and strokes. If you forget everything else, remember this: avoid hydrogenated or partially hydrogenated oils. The companies are clever and hide it; it may say on the label: "0g of trans fats"; however, what they do is increase the serving size to get it under the regulations.

All fats and oils have what's called a "smoke point," a temperature at which the chemical structure deteriorates and forms toxic compounds. When you reach the smoke point, oils turn rancid, and eating foods fried in rancid oil causes increased oxidative stress on our bodies, leading to things like glucose intolerance, protein malfunction, hypertension, and high cholesterol.

Most oils in which the fried food are cooked are obtained from genetically modified plants. One of the top five genetically modified foods used is soy, which is used in meat patties in the United States. The GMO foods can cause digestive issues and some birth defects.

Fried foods are high in saturated fat, which will increase the risk of heart diseases and cause strokes. Most of the fried fast foods contain hundreds of calories, are usually highly processed, and have chemical additives. To increase the shelf life of the food, they are injected with chemical additives that remove nutrients, so fried food is no good for us and doesn't increase our life span.

The fried meat in restaurants is probably polluted or infected with growth hormones that are frequently used to increase the growth speed of livestock. The people who eat fried meat are more vulnerable to certain cancers and infertility. Many people have developed these diseases, according to research.

When oil is reused over and over again, as it often is in fast food chains, the oil continues to break down every time it is heated. It is not only the oil that undergoes a serious change. Other nutrients can be altered by the heating process. An example of this is carbohydrates, which, when heated to very high temperatures, can release a particular type of carcinogen. This is another reason to keep in mind that fast food chains are not the place to find nutrition.

Some fried foods are sterilized with radiation or artificial chemicals. They use inexpensive sterilization methods. Because these methods are cheap, they are often unsafe for consumers' well-being.

For similar measures, a large grilled chicken breast has about 105 calories, but the same chicken breast that is fried comes in at a whopping 323 calories!

Do you still want that fried food we love so much? I know you do, but please say no!

CHAPTER FIVE

CAN I GET SOME SUGAR?

Sugar is very addictive. Sugar is the reason our favorite snacks are hard to pass up and are no good for you. Sugar is in everything; mustard, ketchup, mayonnaise, and just about everything you consume from a restaurant or fast food joint is loaded with tons of sugar and salt.

In a clinical test, researchers introduced mice to cocaine, heroin, and sugar, and the mice preferred the sugar over the cocaine and heroin. Sugar has a devastating effect on the body and mind because it's addictive.

Sugar consumption is out of control. We are taking in 130 pounds of added sugar yearly—that's about 22 teaspoons a day, way over the max set by the American Heart Association in 2009. Science shows that this overload of sugar is stemming from hard-to-detect, hidden added sugars, which are affecting our bodies in all sorts of ways.

Sugar can make our organs fat. Fructose is a component of table sugar and high-fructose corn syrup. Added sugars trigger our liver to store fat more effectively and in weird places. Over time, a diet high in fructose could lead to fat buildup around the liver, resulting in fatty liver disease.

Sugar primes our body for diabetes. Studies show that every extra 150 calories from sugar gives us a 1.1 percent chance of being diagnosed with diabetes.

But just giving up the usual suspects, like sugar, candy bars, and sugary sweeteners, will not do the trick. We have to look for places where manufacturers sneak in hidden sugar. Take a look at these examples of typical hidden-sugar quantities:

- Whole-grain bread: 5 g

- Barbecue sauce : 13 g

- Pasta sauce: 12 g

- Energy drinks: 32 g

- Energy bars: 22 g

- Whole-grain cereal: 18 g

- Soy milk: 10 g

- Frozen entrées: 24 g

- Granola: 20 g

- Granola bars: 12 g

- Flavored oatmeal: 14 g

- Flavored yogurt: 20 g

- Canned baked beans: 12 g

Added sugar is everywhere; we just have to read the labels.

Sugar is the number-one cause of death among people with type 2 diabetes, accounting for 65 percent of deaths.

You should follow the American Heart Association's recommended daily sugar levels, which are five teaspoons (20 g) for women, nine teaspoons (36 g) for men, and three teaspoons (12 g) for children. To give an example of how little sugar that is, one can of soda contains 12 g of sugar, whereas a single slice of whole wheat bread contains up to two teaspoons of that sugar.

Too much sugar is a quick way to get high blood pressure, and I am sure you are not looking to acquire high blood pressure, but this is what happens. Added sugars cause excessive insulin in the bloodstream, which takes its toll on the body's circulatory system and arteries. Chronic high insulin levels cause the smooth muscle cells around each blood vessel to grow faster than normal; this causes tense artery walls, something that puts us on the path to high blood pressure and, ultimately, makes a stroke or heart attack more likely.

Remember, if it's processed, it's not for us. Here's what is done to make whole-grain products. When creating whole-grain flour, wheat kernels are shattered to dust, which, when eaten, causes glucose spikes in our bodies, similar to eating table sugar, white flour, or high-fructose corn syrup.

Sugar will increase our cholesterol.

A study in the Journal of American Medical Association found that after excluding people with high cholesterol, diabetes and people who were highly overweight, the remainder ate the highest levels of added sugar experienced the biggest spikes in bad cholesterol levels, unhealthy triglyceride blood fats, and the lowest good HLD (high-density lipoproteins) cholesterol levels. One theory is that a sugar overload could cause our liver to turn out more bad cholesterol while also inhibiting our body's ability to clean it out.

Sugar triggers the release of chemicals that set off the brain's pleasure center, opioids, and dopamine. People develop a tolerance for sugar, meaning they need more sugar for a "feel-good fix." In rat studies looking at sugar addiction, when animals binge on the sweet stuff, they experience chattering teeth, tremors, shakes, and anxiety when it's taken away.

Prevention advisor Andrew Weil M.D. urges people to be patient as they embark on a diet that cuts added sugars. He says it usually takes about a week for the taste buds to habituate to a lower overall level of sweetness in the diet. After that, foods you used to love may seem sickeningly sweet.

Sugar also increases our cravings; it makes us eat more than we would want to or need to. We cannot put down the fork or spoon when we have a dish prepared with a lot of added sugar. Our food becomes a must-have, which makes our waistline expand.

We should not completely avoid sugar. The best way to consume sugar is from natural fruits that will provide us with plenty of sugar with no harmful effects, and our bodies will thank us.[8]

---

[8] 11 Weird Things Sugar's Doing To Your Body : 4. Sugar ... (n.d.). Retrieved from http://www.prevention.com/food/healthy-eating-tips/weird-effects-sugars-having-o

CHAPTER SIX

THE BIG BANG! A TRANSITION TO A HEALTHY DIET

Transitioning to a healthy diet will lower our blood pressure, control our diabetes, and help prevent cancer and many other conditions while also giving us energy.

When we want to transition into a healthy lifestyle, the first thing we should do is detox the body. A water-only fast works; however, we know this is not where most of us will or would want to start. We should take this journey at our own pace.

Since I have been a practicing vegan for 20 years, I wanted to see what it was like to be on a water-only fast for 21 days. I studied what to do, and I jumped into my first water-only fast; believe it or not, I enjoyed it. The first four days were challenging, but after the fifth day I was no longer hungry, so it became easier for me. I did get a little weak, but fortunately, I could stay home because I had a water filter to supply plenty of clean water.

People who do the water-only fast are advised to consume one to two quarts of pure water or distilled water per day. Although distilled water is not suitable for everyday consumption, it is good during a fast because it increases the ability to bind toxins. The first few days of the fast, as I mentioned earlier, will be the most difficult. Besides the emotional challenge of going without food, the most intense and uncomfortable symptoms of detoxification will arise during these first days. You may get headaches, and in some cases, you will feel sluggish, but don't worry—the body is healing itself.

After we get past the first two or three days, the body goes into a state of ketosis, where it begins to feed itself internally by burning fat cells. Ketosis occurs after around 48 hours for women and 72 hours for men, according to Dr. Joseph Fuhrman, author of *Fasting and Eating for Health*. The length of time we can safely operate in ketosis will vary from person to person. When hunger returns, often called the true hunger, it will be a clear call for nutrition; this is our signal to end the fast.

I was feeling good before I started, but after 21 days, I felt great. I lost a little weight, but overall, the fast helped to restart and reset my body, and my blood pressure was the best it had been in a long time. The body is designed to heal itself, and water fasting is the only fast that helps our body do its job. Water fasting is nothing but pure water, with nothing added to it. The most incredible things happen on the water fast. For one, we will see our bodies heal; the soreness you had in your body will just disappear. Something as simple as acne will go away. Water fasting is incredible, but it's not for everyone, so you should check with your doctor if you are having medical issues.

There are some excellent centers, like the TrueNorth Health Center, which was founded in 1984 by two doctors, Alan Goldhamer and Jennifer Marano. The integrative medicine approach they established offers participants the opportunity to obtain evaluation and treatment for a wide variety of problems. The staff at the TrueNorth Health Center includes medical doctors, osteopaths, chiropractors, naturopaths, psychologists, research scientists, and other health professionals. The center is now the largest facility in the world that specializes in medically supervised water-only fasting.

We can also detox our bodies by changing our diets, but first, we need to change our minds. We need to think about what's important to us; then it becomes easier to change what we eat. Changing what we consume will change our bodies and restore our health.

Health can be restored and or maintained by eating nutritionally, frugally, and pleasurably. First, cut out all animal products, sugars, dairy products, white bread, bakery products, carbonated drinks, hamburgers, hot dogs, snack foods, canned or processed foods, salts and other strong condiments, coffee, ice cream, alcohol, and cigarettes.

Cut down on the size of your meals and combine your foods correctly. Add cooked sprouts, grains, and vegetables to your diet and cut down on your total protein intake. If you have no experience with fasting, skip breakfast several times a week. After eating an improved diet for a month, fast on water or fruit one day a week. Improvements in our living habits, elimination of the worst foods, and increasing our intake of live foods should be our major concerns. We also need to cut down on stress. Get the stress out; if something is stressful, we do not need it.

If we want to change our lives, now is the time to do it. There is no better time than this moment, but we have to make a decision that this is the right thing for us. Don't worry about people who are going to ask, "What are you doing, and why are you doing this?" Your mother or your father may be wondering, "Is this another crazy idea of yours? Why would you give up meat? We've always eaten meat." Making a choice to go plant-based is a personal decision, a decision only you can make and something you should persist with, because if you do, you will be much happier. You will save yourself, help save the planet, and save animals.

When we decide to go plant-based, we have to be careful not to fall into the refined carbs trap. This is the stage in which we start eating a lot of junk food such as bagels, chips, giant pretzels, and vegan junk food. Refined foods are everywhere, but this stuff is not healthy, and it will make us feel worse in the long run. I was an unhealthy vegan for many years, so trust me, I know.

The best way to start is to keep it simple—the "Keep it simple, stupid" (KISS) approach—so that is what I want you to do. Start with fruits, vegetables, salads and experiment with dressings that are homemade, and make sure they are healthy. Try to remove all oils from your diet, if you can. I know I am asking you to give up a lot, but you will get a lot in return, so again, keep it simple at first. Make simple, healthy meals for yourself. I know you are saying, "This is boring!" But before long, you will feel good, and you will understand why boring is great.

By keeping it simple, we are retraining our body to recognize and want healthy food. Before you know it, an organic tomato plucked from our garden will taste incredibly great.

You should invest in some vegan cookbooks; the investment you make will pay off many times over with good health, good looks, and you feeling the best you have felt in a long time. Your body will be running like a racecar with all cylinders firing. Men will not need a little blue pill or any enhancements to perform their duties, no matter how old you are.

Fruits and vegetables do not have to be boring; on the contrary, not only can they be enjoyed for all their essential flavors, but they are also masters of deception and can be used in so many ways. For example, whip up an avocado sauce to blend with your pasta, but not the pasta you are thinking about; you can take zucchini and cut it up into pasta-like strips and make a healthy refreshing dish, but you are still keeping it simple. I have included some jazzy recipes in this book that will help you jazz up your fruit and veggies.

Just because we do not want to eat things that once roamed about doesn't mean we have to sacrifice the pleasures of cooking and eating. With the right ingredients, a vegan plant-based diet can be as sumptuous as any other.

The items listed below fall into three basic categories: 1) Ingredients that can stand in for their animal-based counterparts, 2) Ingredients to enhance plant-based dishes, and 3) Ingredients to add nutrients that a vegan diet may be lacking. This list is in no way complete, but it is a fantastic place to start.

When first transitioning to a plant-based diet, you may feel the need to add fake animal products to your meal plan. That is fine if it helps you step away from the beef, but in general, many of these items are highly processed—glorified vegan junk food—and you may be better off without them. I have listed some of the better products here; just be aware, and take a look at the ingredients list when shopping. You can make a healthy seitan (wheat-based meat substitute) at home I have included recipes and videos at my website: www.jamesjazzyjordan.com.

DAIRY

- ALTERNATIVE MILKS: Almond, soy, rice or hemp milk. I use almond milk.

- BUTTERY SPREAD: Look for non-hydrogenated versions like Earth Balance. I try to stay away from any buttery spreads.

- DAIRY-FREE CHEESE: Daiya cheese melts, and it does not taste like plastic. Eat it as clean as you can, so do not overdo it.

- CREAM CHEESE: Tofutti makes a reasonable mock cream cheese. Do not overdo it. We can make all of these cheese products with nuts.

- SOUR CREAM: Again, Tofutti. Do not overdo it.

- SOY YOGURT: Good for probiotics.

PROTEIN

- TOFURKEY: For those who cannot live without a "roast," my first choice is Field Roast; I think it is the best.

- FIELD ROAST PRODUCTS: Grain-based faux meat products are not too processed and unusually tasty.

- TOFU: Silken tofu for smoothies and puddings; medium or firm tofu for cooking.

- TEMPEH: Soybean-based meat substitute.

- SEITAN: Meat substitute made from wheat gluten. It has a great texture and is a great protein. You can make it yourself. It's easy: if you can make bread, you can make seitan.

- FROZEN VEGETABLE BURGERS: Making your own is better, but these are convenient in a pinch.

- EDAMAME: Fresh (or frozen) soy beans are a great high-protein snack or side.

- BEANS: Dried and home-cooked foods are cheap and are the healthiest options. Get yourself an Instant Pot and cook dry beans without soaking them in 30 minutes.

- CHICKPEAS: Versatile and very tasty.

- SEEDS: Sesame, sunflower, poppy, pumpkin, and chia seeds are all high in protein and healthy fats.

- NUTS: Because they provide protein.

- NUT BUTTERS: Peanut and almond butter.

- CASHEWS: Can be soaked and used in many ways.

GRAINS

- BROWN RICE: Ditch the white rice for more-nutritious brown rice.

- QUINOA: One of the few plant-based perfect proteins.

- STEEL-CUT OATS: Good for breakfast.

- WHOLE GRAIN GRITS: Filling and delicious.

- WHOLE-WHEAT COUSCOUS: More nutritious than regular couscous. Make sure it is a whole food.

- MULTIGRAIN PASTA: Whole-wheat or legume mixes offer more nutrients, and not all of them taste like cardboard.

- SPROUTED BREAD AND TORTILLAS: Food for Life products are nutrient-rich and altogether lovely.

COOKING

- AGAR-AGAR: A vegan substitute for gelatin.

- NUTRITIONAL YEAST: A must for vitamin B12 and very palatable; use like parmesan cheese.

- MISO PASTE: Excellent for adding umami to vegetables. A great anchovy substitute.

- VEGETABLE BROTH: Go for organic, and watch the sodium.

- VEGETABLE BOUILLON: The product Better Than Bouillon No Chicken Base works well.

- TOMATO PASTE: Great (surprising) source of iron.

- DRIED MUSHROOMS: Such as porcini. Adds a meaty component to soups and stews.

- SUNDRIED TOMATOES: Fantastic for adding texture and flavor.

- CAPERS: Great for adding a punch of flavor.

BAKING

- Ener-G Egg Replacer

- FLAX SEEDS: A viable egg substitute for baking.

- CHIA SEEDS: Nutritious pudding and egg substitute.

- VITAL WHEAT GLUTEN: A great binder that also adds protein.

- AGAVE SYRUP: Instead of honey.

- MAPLE SYRUP: Instead of honey.

- BLACKSTRAP MOLASSES: A fantastic source of iron.

CONDIMENTS

- MAYONNAISE: Vegenaise tastes most like traditional mayo; Spectrum is a bit sweeter.

- BRAGG LIQUID AMINOS: Liquid protein concentrate, delicious soy-sauce taste.

- SRIRACHA: Or other favorite hot chili sauces.

- HARISSA: A Tunisian hot pepper paste that makes anything taste good.

- TAHINI: A sesame paste that can be used as a condiment or in preparing Middle Eastern recipes.

- KIMCHI: A cabbage dish. Great source of probiotics, especially if you do not like soy yogurt.

- SAUERKRAUT: Another cabbage dish. A surprising source of health benefits.

When we are shopping for fruits and vegetables, we have to be careful with pesticides. So, the EWG (Environmental Working Group) has provided a list of the top 12 dirty produce, in other words, the ones that are most polluted with pesticides. You should always try to buy the Dirty Dozen™ in organic form, if you can. If you cannot buy organic, it's okay to go for the Clean Fifteen™ (a list of produce with low pesticide residue).

Dirty Dozen™

strawberries	celery	tomatoes
apples	grapes	bell peppers
nectarines	cherries	cherry tomatoes
peaches	spinach	cucumbers

Clean Fifteen™

avocado	onion	eggplant
corn	asparagus	grapefruit
pineapple	mango	cantaloupe
cabbage	papaya	cauliflower
sweet peas	kiwifruit	

CHAPTER SEVEN

You Can Pay Me Now, or You Can Pay Me Later: The Best Food Choices for a Healthy Life

Plant-based living is a lifestyle, not a fad diet; if you change your way of thinking, you will live a healthier and longer life. If you can eat as much as you desire and never have to worry about going hungry again, this is not a diet; it's a lifestyle.

You can throw out all the thoughts of being hungry or not getting enough to eat, but you will have more food than you might think that you can eat.

Eat only when you are hungry, which is after the previous meal has left the stomach. Eat no snacks between meals. Have a small or no breakfast. Eat the biggest meal at noon, when the sun activity is strongest, because solar vibrations aid digestion. Eat a small meal as dinner before sunset if possible, this will give you a longer time to fast our body, before your next meal.

Approach your meal with love and a grateful attitude; bring a peaceful mind to your meals. Do not argue or rush. Enjoy the sound of birds singing and brooks flowing, or peaceful silence. Enjoy your food, eat it slowly, and chew every mouthful thoroughly, reducing to fluid before swallowing. Breathe long and deep with each mouthful.

You should not watch television or read a book; you should focus on your food. Drink at least 20 minutes before or two hours after a meal. Eat one food per meal or combine food correctly for best digestion. Eat juicy foods before substantial foods. Eat raw foods before cooked foods. Stop eating before you feel full, and eat no more than 20 ounces at a single meal.

To avoid pesticides and other poisons, it's best to grow your garden or purchase locally from an organic farm or a reputable natural-food store. One can grow food even in a small apartment: Follow this link to find 44 indoor garden and planter ideas that are very successful and easy to create. For exceptional health, grow an organic garden wherever you are; it can be done in any room. Sprouting greens indoors can reduce the cost of an organic food diet by 50 percent. In your indoor garden, you can grow all the necessary food for winter or summer—at least 70 percent of it.

From organically grown seeds, you can grow sprouts and salad greens to provide a varied menu. Sprouts and greens at an early stage of growth are the most alive foods available. They are still growing at the dinner table. Although raw food is best, those who are not ready for an entirely raw diet may add raw sprouts to cooked dishes just before serving. Eating this way will soon result in substantial improvement to your health.

Unsprouted seeds are hard and have a high starch content, undesirable as food unless they are cooked and seasoned. Sprouting converts the seeds into beneficial food in a period of three to seven days. Why should you eat sprouted beans and seeds?

Sprouted beans and seeds are a great source of protein, and sprouts have more Vitamin C and B, thiamine, niacin, and riboflavin compared to the unsprouted seeds. Beans are also excellent sources of dietary fiber, which helps with the transition of food through the stomach. Sprouts are wonderful for our health. We can buy sprouts, or you can grow our own, and there are excellent examples on YouTube of how you can sprout your seeds and beans.

Here is what the USDA has to say about eating your greens[9]:

"Eating vegetables provides health benefits—people who eat more vegetables and fruits as part of an overall healthy diet are likely to have a reduced risk of some chronic diseases. Vegetables provide nutrients vital for health and maintenance of your body."

Leafy greens are most nutritious when young and tender. The best way to eat them is raw, but you can also steam or sauté them. However, whatever you do, do not overcook them. We will get into some great recipes in later chapters.

Seasonal fruit is best when it is tree or vine ripened. Fruit loses nutrition when over-ripened or under-ripened; the fruit's acid can erode tooth enamel. Fruit is a must in our diet, so have three servings daily.

Beans are a great choice for protein, and I try to eat at least a cup a day. It's funny—they used to say that an apple a day keeps the doctor away, which is true, but if you eat your apples, greens, and beans, I do not think you will have to worry about your physician.

We talked about oils earlier, but I would like to emphasize the point one more time to stay away from oil if you can. If you have to ingest oil, make sure that it's cold-pressed from organically grown produce.

The reason I suggest you stay away from oil is because it is made up of empty calories with no added flavor. The only thing you are getting from oil is additional calories that you do not need.

---

[9] Nutrients and health benefits | Choose MyPlate. (n.d.). Retrieved from https://www.choosemyplate.gov/vegetables-nutrients-health

Junk Foods Disguised as "Health Foods."

1. **Processed "Low-Fat" and "Fat-Free" Foods**
    These are just a bunch of sugar; put back the fat, and keep the sugar out.
    The words "low-fat" or "fat-free" on a packaging usually mean that it is a highly processed product that is loaded with sugar.

2. **Most Commercial Salad Dressings**
    Many salad dressings are loaded with unhealthy ingredients, like sugar, vegetable oils, and trans fats, along with a bunch of artificial chemicals.

3. **Fruit Juices . . . Are Basically Just Liquid Sugar**
    Fruit juice is like fruit, except with all the good stuff (like the fiber) taken out. The main thing left of the actual fruit is the sugar.

4. **"Heart Healthy" Whole Wheat**
    Most "whole wheat" products are not made from whole wheat.
    The grains have been pulverized into very fine flour, making them raise blood sugar just as fast as their refined counterparts.
    There are also studies showing that modern wheat may cause inflammation and increased cholesterol levels, at least when compared to the older varieties.

5. **Cholesterol-Lowering Phytosterols**
    Studies have shown that despite lowering cholesterol levels, phytosterols have adverse effects on the cardiovascular system and may even increase the risk of heart disease and death.

6. **Margarine**
    Back in the day, margarine used to be high in trans fats. These days, it has fewer trans fats but is still loaded with refined vegetable oils.
    Margarine is not food; it is an assembly of chemicals and refined oils that have been made to look and taste like food.
    Recommending trans-fat-laden margarine instead of natural butter may just be the worst nutrition advice in history.

7. **Sports Drinks**

Sports drinks were designed with athletes in mind. These drinks contain electrolytes (salts) and sugar, which can be useful for athletes in many cases. However, most regular people do not need any additional salts, and they certainly have no need for liquid sugar. It is important to stay hydrated, especially around workouts, but most people will be better off sticking to plain water.

8. **Low-Carb Junk Foods**

Food manufacturers have brought various low-carb "friendly" processed foods to the market. This includes highly processed junk foods like the Atkins bars. If you take a look at the ingredients list, you see that there is no real food in there, just chemicals and highly refined ingredients.

These products can be consumed occasionally without compromising the metabolic adaptation that comes with low-carb eating. However, they do not nourish your body. Even though they are technically low-carb, they are still unhealthy.

9. **Agave Nectar**

The problem with agave is that it is no better than sugar. In fact, it is much, much worse. One of the main problems with sugar is that it has excessive amounts of fructose, which can cause severe metabolic problems when consumed in excess. Whereas sugar is about 50 percent fructose and high-fructose corn syrup, about 55 percent of agave contains even more—between 70 and 90 percent. Therefore, gram for gram, agave is even worse than regular sugar. See, "natural" doesn't always equal healthy, and whether agave should even be considered natural is debatable.

10. **Vegan Junk Foods**

There are many processed vegan foods on the market, often sold as convenient replacements for non-vegan foods; vegan bacon is one example.

However, it is important to keep in mind that these are usually highly processed, factory-made products that are bad for just about anyone, including vegans.

11. Brown Rice Syrup

Brown rice syrup contains no refined fructose, just glucose. The absence of refined fructose is good, but rice syrup has a glycemic index of 98, which means that the glucose in it will spike blood sugar extremely fast. Rice syrup is also highly refined and contains almost no essential nutrients. In other words, it is full of "empty" calories. Some concerns have been raised about arsenic contamination in this syrup, another reason to be extra careful with this sweetener.

There are better sweeteners out there, including low-calorie sweeteners like stevia, erythritol, and xylitol, which have some health benefits.

12. Processed Organic Foods

Unfortunately, the word "organic" has become just like any other marketing buzzword. Food manufacturers have found all sorts of ways to make the same junk, except with ingredients that happen to be organic. This includes ingredients like organic raw cane sugar, which is 100 percent identical to regular sugar. It is still just glucose and fructose, with little to no nutrition.

Processed foods that happen to be labeled organic are not necessarily healthy. Always check the label to see what's inside.

13. Vegetable Oils

Bottles of vegetable oil, such as soybean oil, canola oil, grapeseed oil, and many others, have been shown to lower blood cholesterol levels, at least in the short term. However, it is important to keep in mind that blood cholesterol is a risk factor, not a disease in itself. Even though vegetable oils can improve a risk factor, there is no guarantee that they will help prevent actual hard endpoints like heart attacks or death, which is what counts. In fact, several controlled trials have shown that, despite lowering cholesterol, these oils can increase the risk of death from both heart disease and cancer. Avoiding all oils is the safe way to go.

14. Gluten-Free Junk Foods

According to a 2013 survey[10], about a third of people in the U.S. are actively trying to avoid gluten. Many experts think this is unnecessary, but the truth is that gluten, especially from modern wheat, can be problematic for many people.

Not surprisingly, the food manufacturers have brought all sorts of gluten-free foods to the market. The problem with these foods is that they are usually just as bad as the gluten-containing counterparts, if not worse. These are highly processed foods that are very low in nutrients and often made with refined starches that lead to spikes in blood sugar.

So, choose foods that are naturally gluten-free, like plants, and not gluten-free processed foods. Gluten-free junk food is still junk food.

15. Most Processed Breakfast Cereals

When you look at the ingredients list, you see that it is almost nothing but refined grains, sugar, and artificial chemicals. Rule of thumb, if the packaging of food says that it is healthy, then it probably isn't.

The truly healthy foods are those that don't need any health claims, the whole single-ingredient foods. Real food does not need an ingredients list because real food is the ingredient.

---

[10] "Health Foods" That Are Really Junk Foods in Disguise. (n.d.). Retrieved from https://authoritynutrition.com/15-health-foods-that-are-really-junk-foods/

CHAPTER EIGHT

Do You Want Food to Give You Life or Death?

There is an excellent film from the Heart & Stroke Foundation on YouTube titled *Make Health Last. What will your last 10 years look like?* It breaks down what the final ten years of your life could look like; it shows a healthy life or a sick one. If you get a chance, please view it for yourself.

The best food choices come straight from nature; if you can pick it off a tree or a bush and it's naturally ripe, then you have the best the Earth has to offer. We only want to eat what nature provides. Not all foods that you see are straight from nature; some have been modified, such as carrots. You want to avoid blended foods.

There are so many varieties of fruits and vegetables available that you could eat fruits and veggies the rest of your life and never try them all.

There is more nutrition in raw food than cooked, but it is not important to me whether you eat raw or cooked, as long as you are eating healthy food.

It sounds like a crazy question to ask whether you want dead food or live food in your body, but more than 90 percent of the human population chooses to put something dead in their bodies as opposed to living food.

When you consume dead food, you will be tired, achy, irritable, and poorly focused. You may experience high blood pressure and high cholesterol.

Some foods are life-promoting, and some foods are death-promoting. America, like other industrialized nations, has become expert at stripping foods of their natural fiber (where the health-promoting benefits are found) and tarnishing them with synthetic chemicals to turn them from real food into poisonous chemicals. The manipulated foods, sold in packages labeled with promises of good health, contain little, if any, nutrition.

We should eat to help our metabolism, and the best food to do this is real live food. The trillions of cells, bacteria, yeasts, viruses and fungi in the body can be either healthy or unhealthy. The key is not to get rid of the microbes that are found in our mouths, sinuses, eyes, toes, nails, ears, urinary tract, digestive tract, and elsewhere but to provide the proper nutrients to keep all the microbes happy and well balanced.

When we eat dead food, we kill off millions of beneficial probiotics, crippling the natural defenses we need for a healthy immune system.

The Standard American Diet (SAD) is not well balanced, and you do yourself no favors by following it. Choose instead to eat a diet that consists primarily of foods as close to their natural state as possible. That means we are saying goodbye to packages, cans, bags, and boxes for the most part. Real, fresh, local, seasonal, and organic are words that should come to mind when you think of live foods.

When we consume living foods, the enzymes in the foods comingle with our digestive enzymes in a beautiful way—the way they were meant to mingle. There is no battle, no inflammation, and no irritation. The body recognizes the substance as food and knows what to do with it.

CHAPTER NINE

"SPICE OF LIFE"
HOW TO SEASON YOUR FOOD
FOR SUCCESS

Fresh, organically grown foods are high in flavor and a delight to the palate. You can learn to enjoy them without seasoning. Inorganic salt is not food; it is not utilized by the body. Some of it is retained, causing stiffness of the joints, arthritis, hardening of the arteries, and kidney disease. Eating grains induces a craving for salt. A high enough concentration of salt inhibits cell metabolism, eventually causing cell death. While trying to reduce the concentration of salt, your body will retain an excess amount of water in its tissues.

Sea salt, Himalayan salt or tamari miso, which consists of fermented seeds and salt, may be substituted for supermarket salt and should be used sparingly.

Vegetable seasoning, or broth powder, is a substitute for salt. However, be careful when choosing one; it sometimes contains artificial coloring, flavoring, and fillers of brewer's yeast and soybeans, which might combine poorly with other foods.

Seaweed is the best choice for a salty taste. Kelp is a good protective food; it contains all the trace minerals from the sea and has been shown to prevent absorption of strontium-90 into the body. Sea vegetables are a good choice, but with the toxic waste in Japan, make sure you know where they were harvested.

Garlic, cayenne, chili, and ginger root are noted for healing qualities when one is eating a cooked-food diet. They provide flavor for the transitional diet. However, once the body is detoxed, they can act as irritants to the kidneys, liver, and mucous lining of the digestive tract.

Bottom line: Try to stay away from a lot of salt as much as possible. The best way to get your salt taste is from kelp, herbs, and spices.

CHAPTER TEN

Belly Fat Is a Killer . . . Yes, I am Talking to You

On your body, there's one place where fat is especially dangerous. Fat around the midsection is a high-risk factor for heart disease, type 2 diabetes, and even some types of cancers. Most studies show this to be true. The tests show that too much belly fat tends to prompt a loss of sensitivity to insulin, which is a crucial hormone that helps the body burn energy. When insulin loses its power, the body responds by pumping out more of the hormone, which only throws the system off balance further.

As a result, belly fat brings on a whole cascade of problems known as insulin-resistance syndrome or metabolic syndrome. Over 50 million Americans are affected—big bellies come with a frightening array of potential complications. For one thing, people with insulin resistance often develop type 2 diabetes. They also tend to have high blood pressure and bad cholesterol, which, according to numerous studies, are a recipe for heart disease.

Check your belly fat with a tape measure. These numbers will tell you if you have a problem. If you are a man, a waist circumference of more than 40 inches means you are at a higher risk for heart disease and many other diseases. Women with a waist circumference of over 35 inches are at increased risk.

In general, our body shape is a reflection of both our genes and our lifestyle. Different people put on fat in different places. Some people naturally carry weight in their midsections (an apple shape) while others are more bottom-heavy (a pear shape).

Inactivity or a sedentary lifestyle is not the only reason; it's the food you are consuming. Put down the fast food, beer, and soda. Stress—such as dissatisfaction that comes from a high-pressure, low-paying job—can encourage the buildup of fat around the midsection.

A bulge in the belly is a wake-up call. If you can trim down your midsection, you will go a long way toward preventing the health problems associated with belly fat. A healthy lifestyle can ward off fat from top to bottom, and especially the middle. When you lose weight, your body will make getting rid of belly fat the highest priority.

Cosmetic surgeons cannot help us; we have to change our lifestyle. It's all about what we are eating, drinking, and doing. Looking healthy is not the same as being healthy. Women who had about 30 percent of their body fat suctioned off didn't move any closer to avoiding diabetes or heart disease. Specifically, the procedure did not lower blood pressure or improve their response to insulin. A perfectly flat stomach may not be within your reach, but a healthier body certainly is.

The race to good health is a marathon, not a sprint, so take your time and get it right. Have a happy journey, and remember that health is wealth.

Jazzy's Recipes

We should keep breakfast meals simple; we need to fast our bodies as long as possible so try to eat your last meal between 6 and 7 PM, and then do not eat again until maybe 10 or 11 the next morning. That way our bodies have plenty of time to fast and clean itself out. We should start the day with a small but wholesome meal.

Ideal Breakfast

Drinking juice each day is the easiest way for busy people to get the vegetables they need. Juices make a cleansing, nutritious breakfast or an energizing mid-afternoon snack. Use organically grown produce whenever possible, especially for greens that can't be peeled, such as kale and celery. Energizing, purifying juice and green juices should be our staples since they are the highest in nutrients and lowest in calories and sugars.

Juicers

Juicers are great to have for a healthy life; the Omega 350 HD, is an extremely high-quality low-speed juicer that will help us to get through just about every fruit and vegetable with ease. It has a very small and compact base, so it will not take up much room on the kitchen countertop. It has an extra large spout, so there is not too much chopping. It is quiet and very quick to disassemble and clean.

Blenders

Get a high-speed blender; it can be used to breakdown veggies to juice. The veggies will have to be cut up into 1-inch pieces so not to stall the blender. To make juice from a blender, add fruits and veggies with about half a cup of water and blend until smooth, run the juice through a strainer to get rid of the pulp, or keep the pulp for more fiber. Some people prefer using the blender over the juicer because there is very little fiber when juicing with a juicer. A blender is a must have. If there is a choice to be made between a juicer or blender, I will take the blender; they are so helpful.

Fruit and More Fruit

Fruit is the perfect food. A meal of apples, oranges, plums or pears can be a satisfying treat. Fruit acids do not make the body acid. Rather, they increase the alkalinity of the body.

Selecting Fruit

Watermelon is a favorite because it is very filling, and it also helps us stay hydrated. Watermelon is noted for its alkaline pH and a high predominance of alkaline materials; watermelons are generally at least three times more alkaline than acidic. They are a very rich source of potassium. They are valuable in kidney disorders because they induce diuretic action.

If not watermelon, have organic citric fruit. For a nice pick-me-up have a banana, apple, mango, avocado and papaya smoothie, or just peel and eat whole (which is the best way to have them) because we get the fiber. This combination of fruit will have us energized for the day. This type of breakfast is ideal during the summer. Fruit is quick, easy and healthy.

Available all year round, apples are excellent food; alkalinizing, cleansing, and easy to digest.

Avocado, although rich in minerals and vitamins and containing about 2 percent protein, is about 13.4 percent fat and, therefore, it's difficult to digest. However, it's very delicious and a good source of healthy fat.

Fruit should always be ripe; that is the only way to eat fruit. Unripe fruit is not good for us, and overripe is also no good: it has to be ripe.

When we are making the transition from sugar, it is always nice to have something we can consume that will give us that sweetness. Dried fruit is excellent for a sweet treat. Alternatively, take half of avocado, half a cup of water, eight pitted dates (or two slices of pineapple dried or fresh), and blend, adding more water if needed.

POWER GREENS DRINKS AND SMOOTHIES

Green Drink

* I like the following recipe juiced instead of blended. However, if you blend, be sure to add one and a half cups of water.

- 2 apples
- 3 celery stalks
- 2 handfuls of spinach
- ½ fennel bulb
- 1 cucumber

- 3 romaine lettuce leaves
- 2 kale leaves, stems removed
- 1-inch piece of ginger, peeled
- ½ lemon, peeled

Tangerine Green Smoothie

- 2 tangerines
- 1 green apple
- 1 banana, frozen if possible
- 2 kale leaves, stems removed
- Small handful of spinach

- 1 to 1½ cups water or enough to blend into a smooth texture
- 2 or 3 dates, to sweeten
- Small handful of cilantro
- Ice (optional)

* Blend until smooth.

Banana and Papaya Smoothie

* For quick and easy smoothie take one banana, one cup of papaya, and one cup of apple juice. Blend until smooth.

Wake Up the Third Eye

* Take 1 papaya and the juice of 2 oranges, and blend the papaya and orange juice to a puree. It is an exceptional aid to digestion.

Watermelon-Honeydew Smoothie

* Take 3 cups of watermelon and 1 cup of honeydew melon. Place in blender and push down sides until the melon extracts enough juice to blend on its own. When blended, add 1 cup of ice and blend until thick. Sweetener can be added if desired. Serve in tall glasses with a straw.

Mango-Papaya Smoothie

- 1 mango, diced
- 1 cup papaya, diced
- 1 cup fresh spinach, lightly packed
- ½ cup celery, cubed
- ½ cup ice (optional)
- ¼ cup old-fashioned or quick-cooking rolled oats
- 6 or 7 cashews
- 1 tablespoon fresh ginger, chopped

1. Put all the ingredients in a blender and process on high speed until smooth.

2. Pour into a tall glass and serve immediately. For a thicker smoothie, add more cashews.

Banana-Kale Smoothie

- 1 cup unsweetened pineapple juice
- 1 ripe banana
- 1 kale leaf
- ½ cup celery, cubed
- ½ cup ice (optional)
- ¼ cup old-fashioned or quick-cooking rolled oats
- 6 or 7 toasted pecans

Cantaloupe Smoothie

1. Using 2 small cantaloupes, cut the cantaloupe in half crosswise.

2. Using a spoon, scoop out the seeds and discard.

3. Scoop out the flesh of the cantaloupe and place it in a blender; process on medium speed until smooth.

4. Serve immediately.

Berry Smoothie

- ¼ cup water
- 1 cup fresh or frozen strawberries, blueberries, or blackberries
- 1 ripe banana, fresh or frozen

1. To make it a frosty smoothie, use frozen fruit.

2. Place all the ingredients in a blender and process on medium speed until smooth.

3. Serve immediately.

Piña Colada Smoothie

- 1 ripe banana, fresh or frozen
- ½ orange, peeled and sectioned
- ½ cup chopped fresh pineapple

1. Place all the ingredients in a blender and process on medium speed until smooth.
2. Serve immediately.

Veggie Juice

- 2 celery stalks
- 1 small ripe tomato, cut into quarters
- 1 red bell pepper, cut into pieces
- 1 cucumber, cut into pieces
- 10 parsley and/or cilantro sprigs
- 1 garlic clove
- ½ teaspoon fresh lemon juice
- Dash of cayenne or hot sauce (optional)

* This juice has a great taste with all the vitamins needed.

Tropical Fruit Salad

- 1 ripe mango, or ½ small ripe papaya, cubed
- ½ ripe banana, sliced
- 1 kiwifruit, peeled and sliced
- ½ cup raspberries or sliced strawberries
- ¼ cup orange-maple cream sauce

1. Combine the mango, banana, kiwifruit, and berries in a small bowl and toss gently with a spoon.
2. Serve immediately, plain or with orange maple cream sauce.

Here how to make an orange-maple cream sauce:

- ½ cup maple syrup
- ¼ cup chopped orange peel
- ½ cup orange juice
- Pinch of salt

* Combine all the ingredients. Let the mixture stand over hot, not boiling, water for about 30 minutes to blend flavors.

Breakfast—Quick and Healthy

Apple-Orange Oatmeal

- 8 cups unsweetened apple juice
- Grated zest and juice of 1 orange
- ½ cup raisins
- 1 teaspoon ground cinnamon
- ½ teaspoon ground nutmeg
- 4 cups quick-cooking rolled oats (not instant)

1. Put the apple juice, orange zest, and juice, raisins, cinnamon, and nutmeg in a large saucepan and stir to combine.

2. Bring to a boil over high heat. Add the oats and stir rapidly for 30 seconds.

3. Cover, decrease the heat to low and cook for 5 minutes.

4. Serve hot.

Apple-Cherry Oatmeal

* Substitute the orange zest and juice with 3 apples, peeled, cored, and diced, and the raisins with a half cup of dried cherries.

Pineapple-Coconut Oatmeal

* Replace the apple juice with 8 cups of unsweetened pineapple juice, and replace the raisins with 2 cups of unsweetened shredded dried coconut.

Berries and Almond Cream

- 1 cup mixed berries (such as blackberries, blueberries, berries, raspberries, or sliced strawberries)
- 1 teaspoon pure maple syrup
- ½ cup almond cream

1. Place the berries and sweetener in a small bowl and toss gently.

2. Transfer to a small dish and top with the almond cream.

3. Serve immediately.

Almond-Sunflower Seed Cereal

- 2 tablespoons soaked raw almonds
- 2 tablespoons soaked raw sunflower seeds
- 1 tablespoon soaked raw walnuts or pecans (optional)
- ½ cup chopped or sliced fresh fruit (such as apple, banana, berries, kiwifruit, mango, peach, or pineapple)
- ½ cup almond milk

1. Combine the almonds, sunflower seeds, optional walnuts, and fruit in a small bowl.

2. Serve immediately with almond milk.

Banana-Blueberry Pancakes

- 2 ripe bananas
- 1 tablespoon maple syrup
- ½ teaspoon cinnamon
- ¾ cup pecans, chopped
- ½ cup blueberries

1. Place bananas in a bowl and gently mash with a fork until large pieces are broken down, but don't make it mushy like baby food.

2. Add remaining ingredients, reserving half of the blueberries.

3. Lightly incorporate ingredients.

4. Use a nonstick dehydrator sheet and divide mixture into 3 or 4 pancakes.

5. Divide remaining blueberries and press on top of pancakes.

6. Dehydrate for 4 hours at 110 degrees Fahrenheit.

7. When dry enough to turn, flip onto mesh screen and use a knife to help separate the pancake from the nonstick sheet if necessary.

8. Dehydrate for another 3 to 4 hours.

9. Pancakes should be soft inside, with a light crust on the outside.

10. If needed right away, it is okay to cook pancakes on the stovetop: Place the formed pancakes into a nonstick frying pan and cook for 2 to 3 minutes on each side.

Quick and Easy Banana and Blueberry Pancakes

- 2 ripe bananas, mashed
- 1 ¼ cups almond milk
- 3 ½ teaspoon baking powder
- 1 teaspoon salt
- 1 tablespoon sugar
- 3 tablespoon vegan "butter," melted
- 1 ½ cups flour
- 1 ½ cups blueberries

1. Combine all the ingredients in a large bowl.
2. Heat the pan.
3. Scoop half a cup of batter onto the pan and wait until bubbles come through the top. When the bottom of the pancake is golden, flip the pancake.
4. When both sides of the pancake are golden, remove from the pan.
5. Repeat until batter is finished.
6. Serve with maple syrup, sliced bananas, and blueberries.

Tofu Scramble

Jazz up this basic recipe by adding 1 cup of chopped vegetables, mushrooms, spinach, or vegan meat.

- 14 ounce (1 packet) firm or extra-firm tofu, drained
- 3 tablespoons nutritional yeast
- 1 tablespoon Dijon mustard
- 1 teaspoon garlic powder
- 1 teaspoon onion powder
- ½ teaspoon turmeric
- ½ teaspoon ground cumin
- 1 cup vegetables, mushrooms, spinach, or vegan meat, chopped (optional)
- Salt and pepper, to taste

1. Place the tofu in non-stick skillet and break apart with a spatula into large chunks.

2. Cook over medium-high heat until the tofu releases its water, about 3 to 4 minutes.

3. Add nutritional yeast, Dijon, garlic powder, onion powder, cumin, and turmeric, stirring to coat evenly.

4. Break up any large remaining chunks of tofu until the tofu is crumbly and looks like scrambled eggs.

5. Continue to cook, stirring regularly, until all water has evaporated (about 10 minutes).

6. If necessary, add a splash of water or non-dairy milk to prevent sticking.

7. If using the vegetables or vegan meat, mix in and continue to cook until everything is thoroughly warmed.

8. Add salt and pepper to taste and serve immediately.

Omelette

- ⅔ cups water
- ⅓ cup chickpea flour
- 1 tablespoons ground flax seeds
- 1 tablespoons nutritional yeast (optional)
- ½ teaspoon baking powder
- ¼ teaspoon black salt (optional but adds egg flavor)
- ¼ teaspoon white pepper
- ⅛ teaspoon turmeric
- ⅛ teaspoon Salt
- ½ teaspoon garlic powder
- ⅛ teaspoon chili flakes (optional)

SUGGESTED TOPPINGS:

* Mushrooms, spinach, chargrilled red peppers, pesto, hummus, potatoes.

French Toast

- 8 slices vegan bread
- 1 cup non-dairy milk
- ¼ cup chickpea flour
- 1 teaspoon ground cinnamon
- 1 teaspoon pure maple syrup
- ½ teaspoon fine salt
- ¼ teaspoon ground nutmeg
- ¼ teaspoon vanilla extract (optional)
- Extra maple syrup for serving

1. Whisk non-dairy milk, flour, cinnamon, maple syrup, salt, nutmeg, and vanilla extract, if using, in a shallow bowl.

2. Dip a few slices into the mixture and transfer to the nonstick skillet. Cook for 3 minutes, flip over and cook for 3 minutes more.

3. Garnish with cinnamon and sliced fresh fruit.

Cinnamon-Banana Toast Crunch

- 2 slices vegan bread
- ¼ cup pure maple syrup
- 1 teaspoon ground cinnamon
- ¼ teaspoon vanilla or banana extract (optional)
- 1 banana
- 2 slices bread, lightly toasted

1. While bread is toasting, whisk the syrup, cinnamon, and extract together or use a mixer.

2. Plate the toast and smear the syrup mixture across both slices of toast, and let it soak in, about 30–60seconds.

3. Top each slice with fresh banana slices and garnish with a light drizzle of pure maple syrup, if desired.

Brown Rice Pancakes

Brown rice flour adds a bit of a crunch and a nice nutty taste to traditional pancakes.

- ½ cup whole-wheat pastry flour
- ½ cup brown rice flour
- 1 tablespoon baking powder
- ½ teaspoon ground cinnamon
- ⅛ teaspoon fine salt
- 1 cup non-dairy milk
- 2 tablespoons pure maple syrup

1. Whisk flours, baking powder, cinnamon, and salt together in a large bowl.

2. Combine non-dairy milk with maple syrup.

3. Pour the wet mixture into the dry and stir until just combined (a few lumps are okay).

4. Let it rest for 10 minutes.

5. Heat skillet over very low heat.

6. Transfer mixture to a large liquid measuring cup, or use greased ¼-cup measuring cup,

7. Pour in ¼ cup of batter into the nonstick skillet.

8. Cook on one side until bubbles form, then gently flip and cook for another 2 to 3 minutes.

Heart-Healthy Sausage Patties

- 2 garlic cloves
- 1 small onion, quartered
- 1 carrot, peeled and cut into large chunks
- ½ teaspoon fennel seeds
- Water, as needed
- 1 can (15-ounces) pinto beans, drained
- 1 tablespoon almond flour or almond meal

- 1 tablespoon nutritional yeast
- 1 teaspoon smoked paprika
- ½ teaspoon dried oregano (1 teaspoon fresh)
- ½ teaspoon dried sage (1 teaspoon fresh)
- ½ teaspoon dried basil (1 teaspoon fresh)
- ½ teaspoon dried thyme (1 teaspoon fresh)
- ½ teaspoon sea salt

1. Preheat the oven to 400 degrees Fahrenheit.

2. Line a baking sheet with a silicone mat or parchment paper.

3. In a food processor, add the garlic, onion, and carrot, and chop until fine (or chop by hand).

4. Place a medium skillet over medium heat.

5. Add the onion-carrot mixture and the fennel seeds.

6. Cook for about 4 minutes, or until the vegetables are soft, adding water if needed.

7. Remove from the heat and cool.

8. In the food processor, add the pinto beans and pulse until roughly chopped, but not to a paste.

9. Add the onion-carrot mixture to the processor and process until blended.

10. Transfer the contents to a medium bowl.

11. Add the almond flour, yeast, paprika, oregano, sage, basil, thyme, and salt.

12. Mix until the ingredients are combined.

13. Measure ¼ cup of sausage and shape into a patty by hand.

14. Carefully place each patty onto the prepared pan.

15. Continue with the remaining sausage.

16. Bake for 25 to 30 minutes, until crispy on the outside but still moist on the inside.

17. Remove from the oven and cool for a few minutes before serving.

Sweet Potato Waffles

- 1 ¼ cups almond flour
- 2 teaspoons baking powder
- ½ teaspoon sea salt
- Dash nutmeg
- Dash cinnamon
- ⅓ cup coconut oil
- 1 ½ cups unsweetened coconut milk
- 1 cup mashed sweet potato
- Cooking spray
- 1 cup unsweetened applesauce

1. Preheat the waffle iron.

2. In a large bowl, combine the almond flour, baking powder, salt, nutmeg, and cinnamon.

3. In a medium bowl, whisk together the coconut oil and coconut milk until combined.

4. Transfer the liquid ingredients to the bowl with the dry ingredients. Whisk until combined.

5. Gently fold the sweet potatoes into the batter, being careful not to over mix.

6. Spray the waffle iron with cooking spray before making each waffle.

7. Make the waffles according to the directions indicated on the waffle iron.

8. Serve each waffle with a quarter cup of applesauce.

Breakfast Fajitas

- 1 bell pepper (any color), cored, seeded, and sliced
- 1 sweet onion, chopped
- 1 cup broccoli florets, cooked
- ½ cup mushrooms, sliced
- 1 cup cherry tomatoes, halved if large
- ½ cup sliced zucchini or other squash
- 2 garlic cloves, peeled and chopped
- 1 jalapeño, chopped (optional)
- 1 teaspoon sea salt
- ½ teaspoon cumin
- 2 tablespoons fresh cilantro
- Juice of ½ lime
- Salsa fresca

1. Spray a large nonstick skillet with cooking spray and place it over medium heat.

2. Add the bell pepper, onion, broccoli, mushrooms, tomatoes, zucchini, garlic, and jalapeño (if using).

3. Cook for about 7 minutes, or until the desired level of tenderness.

4. Add salt, cumin, and cilantro. Cook, for 3 minutes more.

5. Remove from heat and add the lime juice.

6. Divide between two plates and serve with salsa fresca.

Cajun Home Fries

Let me warn you: these fries are addictive!

- 2 medium sweet potatoes, diced
- 2 teaspoons garlic powder
- 2 teaspoons onion powder
- 1 teaspoon onion flakes
- ¼ teaspoon paprika or cayenne pepper
- Salt and pepper to taste

1. Preheat oven to 400 degrees Fahrenheit.
2. Get a parchment paper lined cookie sheet and set aside.
3. Place potatoes in a mixing bowl.
4. Spray with cooking spray and sprinkle spices over the top.
5. Be generous with garlic and onion, but do not use too much cayenne or paprika.
6. Add salt and pepper.
7. Mix to evenly coat.
8. Re-spray and repeat.
9. Transfer to cookie sheet, making sure there is no overlap.
10. Bake for 15 to 25 minutes, or until fully cooked and crisp.

Herbed Home Fries

- 2 medium sweet potatoes, diced
- 2 teaspoons garlic powder
- 2 teaspoons onion powder
- 1 teaspoon Italian seasoning salt to taste

1. Preheat oven to 400 degrees Fahrenheit.

2. Get a parchment paper lined cookie sheet and set aside.

3. Place sweet potatoes in a mixing bowl.

4. Spray with cooking spray and sprinkle spices over the top.

5. Be generous with garlic and onion.

6. Add salt.

7. Mix to evenly coat.

8. Re-spray and repeat.

9. Transfer to cookie sheet, making sure there is no overlap.

10. Bake for 15 to 25 minutes, or until fully cooked and crisp.

Granola

- ½ cup oat groats, soaked for 4 hours or overnight
- ½ cup buckwheat groats, soaked for 4 hours or overnight
- 1 cup almonds, soaked for 4 hours
- 1 cup sunflower seeds, soaked for 2 hours
- 1 cup pumpkin seeds, soaked for 2 hours
- 1 cup pecans, soaked for 2 hours
- 1 ½ cups dates, soaked for 1 hour or until soft
- 1 cup raisins, soaked for 1 hour
- 4 apples, coarsely chopped
- ½ cup blueberries
- 1 teaspoon cinnamon
- 1 tablespoon lemon juice
- ½ cup maple syrup, or sweetener of choice (slightly more if making bars)
- 1 teaspoon maple extract
- Pinch of salt

1. Add groats, nuts, and seeds to food processor and pulse-chop 4 or 5 times, stopping to scrape down sides.

2. Remove the mixture and place in a mixing bowl.

3. Add apples, dates, maple syrup, maple extract, lemon, cinnamon, and salt to food processor and blend until smooth.

4. Remove to mixing bowl and blend in blueberries and raisins.

5. Mix until well incorporated.

6. Spread mixture on a nonstick dehydrator sheet and dehydrate at 110 degrees Fahrenheit for 8 hours.

7. Flip over onto dehydrator sheet and continue dehydrating for another 8 hours or until granola is dry.

8. Test to see if it is crisp by breaking off a small piece.

BREADS and CRACKERS

Caramelized Onion Bread

- 3 cups onion, thinly sliced
- 2 cups sprouted wheatberry, ground in blender (or a spice/coffee grinder)
- 1 cup sunflower seeds, ground in blender (or a spice/coffee grinder)
- ¼ cup maple syrup
- 2 cups zucchini, coarsely chopped
- 3 tablespoons extra-virgin olive oil
- 2 tablespoons sunflower lecithin
- 1 apple, coarsely chopped
- 3 tablespoons nutritional yeast (not raw but vegan)
- 1 cup sundried tomatoes, soaked until soft
- 1 tablespoon lemon juice
- 1 clove garlic
- ½ teaspoon salt
- 1 avocado, chopped

- ¼ cup Irish Moss paste
- 1 cup flaxseed, ground into a meal in your spice or coffee grinder
- ½ cup or more of water, as needed
- 1 teaspoon oregano
- 1 teaspoon thyme
- ½ cup soaked dates
- 2 tablespoons tamari, nama shoyu, or freshly milled pepper to taste

1. Sprinkle onions with salt, stevia, or dry sweetener of choice and let sit for 30 minutes.

2. Drain dates, pit, and place in a high-speed blender with 1 tablespoon tamari, 1 tablespoon water, and a dash of extra-virgin olive oil.

3. Add the date mixture to the onions and mix well.

4. Place onions on a nonstick dehydrator sheet and dehydrate for 2 hours or until soft.

5. Place all remaining ingredients, except onion and flax meal, in food processor.

6. Mix until ingredients are broken down and fluffy (best done in two batches).

7. When all ingredients are well incorporated, and the mixture looks light, remove half and add flax meal to the remaining half.

8. Pulse until flax is incorporated.

9. Place all the dough in a mixing bowl, add caramelized onions and use hands to incorporate.

10. Spread half-inch thick dough onto two nonstick dehydrator sheets.

11. Dehydrate for 8 hours at 105–110 degrees Fahrenheit.

12. When it's dry on top, flip onto mesh dehydrator tray and invert.

13. Peel off the nonstick sheet and continue to dehydrate for approximately 8 to 10 hours, or more, until the bread feels light and crusty on the outside and slightly soft in the center.

Pizza Crackers

- 2 cups flaxseeds soaked in 2 cups of water 4–6 hours
- ¼ cup sundried tomatoes, soaked until soft
- ¼ cup of hemp seeds
- ¼ cup sunflower seeds, ground in a spice or coffee grinder
- ¼ cup pumpkin seeds, ground in a spice or coffee grinder
- ½ cup onion, chopped
- 1 small clove garlic, crushed
- 1 teaspoon extra-virgin olive oil
- Dash of tamari or nama shoyu
- 1 teaspoon lemon juice
- 1 tablespoon Italian seasonings, oregano, rosemary, marjoram, basil
- Himalayan Salt to taste
- Freshly milled pepper to taste
- ¼ cup raw olives, finely chopped
- Water as needed

1. In a food processor, chop all ingredients except olives until smooth.

2. Adjust salt and herbs to taste.

3. Scrape down the sides and add water if needed to smooth out any lumps.

4. Mix in olives by hand.

5. Divide onto 2 or 3 nonstick dehydrator sheets and spread into large squares about an inch thick.

6. Dehydrate for 6 hours at 105 degrees Fahrenheit, then flip and score.

7. Dehydrate another 6 hours or until crisp and dry.

Raw Vegan Carrot and Flax Crackers

The dilemma after juicing, what to do with the pulp?

How about making some easy crackers that are grain-free, gluten-free and flourless!

So just basically put all the pulp in the mixer, add seeds, stir everything and then spread it out over a dehydrator tray and the next day . . . crackers!

- 3 cups organic carrot pulp
- ½ cup organic flax seeds (freshly ground)
- ½ - 1 organic tomato
- 1 organic lemon (freshly juiced)
- ½ cup organic chia seeds
- ½ cup organic sesame seeds
- ¾ cups purified or filtered water

1. Put all ingredients (except sesame seeds and chia seeds) in a mixer and process until well blended.

2. Pour the liquid mixture into a medium-sized bowl and add sesame seeds and chia seeds and stir gently.

3. Spread the mixture onto the Paraflexx lining or parchment paper on a dehydrator tray and spread evenly (not too thin).

4. Dehydrate at 105 degrees Fahrenheit for approximately 10 to 12 hours.

5. Transfer to a mesh tray and continue to dehydrate for an additional 2 to 4 hours or until firm and crisp.

6. Cut into cracker shapes and store in an air-tight container to keep them hard.

7. No more wasted pulp and super nutritious crackers!

Banana Bread

- 1 ¾ cups spelt flour or flour of choice
- 2 teaspoons baking powder
- ½ teaspoon baking soda
- Pinch of mineral salt
- ⅓ cup neutral flavored or warmed coconut oil
- 1 teaspoon vanilla extract
- ⅓ cup organic pure cane sugar or finely chopped dates
- 4 small or 3 large bananas, about 1 ¾ cup (preferably overripe), mashed

1. Preheat oven to 350 degrees Fahrenheit.

2. Combine flour, baking powder, baking soda and salt in a medium or large size bowl and set aside.

3. In a small bowl mix oil, sugar, and vanilla.

4. Combine wet ingredients with dry ingredients and mix briefly, set aside.

5. Mash bananas, add to batter and mix until combined.

6. Pour or spoon into a well-greased loaf pan (I use oil to grease)

7. Bake for 50–60 minutes (use the toothpick test in the center of the loaf; if it comes out clean, it is about ready).

8. Remove from the oven and cool for 10 minutes.

Soups

Comforting Winter Soup

- 1 small bunch kale
- 4 cups vegetable broth, divided
- 1 medium onion, diced
- 4 garlic cloves, minced
- 2 celery stalks, sliced
- 2 large carrots, peeled and sliced
- 1 leek, white parts only, thinly sliced
- 1 tablespoon Italian seasoning or poultry seasoning mix
- 2 bay leaves
- 1 tablespoon mild curry powder
- ¼ teaspoon ground ginger
- Salt and pepper to taste

1. Remove stems from kale and tear into bite-sized pieces and set aside.

2. Line a large pot with 2 cups of broth, and add onion, garlic, celery, carrots, leek, seasoning blend, bay leaves, and curry powder.

3. Bring to a boil over a high heat, and continue to boil until onion is translucent (about 5 minutes).

4. Add remaining broth and reduce the heat to medium.

5. Once boiling, add the kale, constantly stirring until wilted, soft, and incorporated into the soup (about 2 minutes).

6. Remove from the heat, add ginger, then salt and pepper.

7. Remove bay leaves before serving.

Creamy Carrot Soup

- 1 pound carrots, peeled and sliced
- 1 small onion, diced
- ¼ cup instant oats
- ½ cup non-dairy milk
- ½ teaspoon ground ginger
- ¼ teaspoon allspice
- Salt and pepper to taste

1. In a medium saucepan, combine 2 cups of water, carrots, onion, and oats over high heat.

2. Bring to a boil, then reduce the heat to medium.

3. Continue to cook, stirring frequently, until oats are cooked and carrots are fork-tender (about 5 minutes).

4. Transfer to a blender (in batches, if necessary) and combine with non-dairy milk.

5. Blend until smooth and creamy, adding an extra splash of non-dairy milk if needed.

6. Transfer back to the saucepan and stir in ginger and allspice.

7. Gently reheat and add salt and pepper.

Optional: Garnish with chopped scallions and fresh pepper.

African Kale and Yam Soup

- 1 small red onion, thinly sliced
- 2 cups vegetable broth
- 2 cups yams, peeled and diced
- 5 cups kale, torn into bite-sized pieces
- 2 teaspoon chili powder
- 1 teaspoon ground cumin
- 1 teaspoon garlic powder
- ¼ teaspoon red pepper flakes, or to taste
- 1 teaspoon mild curry powder
- 1 tablespoon yellow miso paste
- ¼ teaspoon cinnamon

1. In a medium pot add a quarter cup of water and cook the onion over high heat until translucent (about 3 minutes).

2. Add broth, yams, and three-quarter cup of water and bring to a boil.

3. Once boiling, reduce heat to medium and cook until yams are almost fork-tender (about 3 minutes).

4. Immediately add kale and remaining ingredients.

5. Continue to cook, stirring frequently, until the kale is dark green and soft (about 3 minutes more).

6. Set aside for 5 to 10 minutes, allowing flavors to merge, then serve.

Curried Sweet Potato Soup

- 1 medium sweet potato or yam
- ½ sweet onion, chopped
- 3 garlic cloves, minced
- 1 cup vegetable broth
- ½ to 1 teaspoon mild curry powder
- ¼ to ½ teaspoon garam masala
- ½ cup non-dairy milk
- ¼ cup cooked wild rice

1. Preheat oven to 425 degrees Fahrenheit.

2. Bake the sweet potato until fully cooked (about 45 minutes to 1 hour).

3. Allow potato to cool completely, then peel and discard the skin.

4. Transfer potato to a blender and set aside.

5. In a medium saucepan, combine onion, garlic, broth, a half teaspoon of the curry powder, and a quarter teaspoon of the garam masala.

6. Bring to a boil, then reduce heat to low, cover, and simmer until onion is translucent, about 5 to 7 minutes.

7. Transfer onion mixture to the blender with the potato, add non-dairy milk and blend until smooth and creamy.

8. Return soup to saucepan and heat thoroughly.

9. Taste and adjust seasonings, adding half a teaspoon of the curry or a quarter teaspoon more of the garam masala, if desired.

10. If the soup becomes too thick, thin it out with a little non-dairy milk or water.

11. Ladle soup into bowls, adding warm rice into the center.

12. Sprinkle with ground cinnamon for garnish and serve.

Burgers and Wraps

Black Bean Burgers

A good and quick meal, this burger fits the bill perfectly.

- 1 can (15-ounces) black beans, drained and rinsed
- ¼ cup fresh cilantro, minced
- 1 teaspoon ground cumin
- ½ teaspoon dried oregano
- Cayenne pepper to taste
- Salt and pepper to taste
- Breadcrumbs
- Vegan hamburger buns

1. Preheat oven to 350 degrees Fahrenheit.

2. Grease a cookie sheet or line with parchment paper and set aside.

3. Pulse beans in food processor until mashed well, or mash manually using a potato masher or fork.

4. Transfer to a mixing bowl and stir in cilantro and spices, plus salt and pepper.

5. Add breadcrumbs (about ¼ cup) as necessary until the mixture can be handled and isn't terribly sticky.

6. Shape the mixture into patties.

7. Lightly spray each patty with cooking spray and bake for 7 minutes.

8. Flip, re-spray, and bake for 7 to 10 minutes more—until crisp on the outside and thoroughly warm.

9. Serve immediately on buns.

10. Because there is no oil, these patties dry out easily, so eat them right away.

Mushroom Burgers

The mushrooms naturally add a beefy flavor and hold in moisture.

- 1 slice vegan bread
- 8-ounces cremini mushrooms
- 1 can (15-ounces) pinto or kidney beans, drained
- 1 teaspoon paprika
- 1 teaspoon onion powder
- 1 teaspoon garlic powder
- ⅓ cup vital wheat gluten
- 2 tablespoon soy sauce
- 2 tablespoon steak sauce
- 2 tablespoon BBQ sauce

1. Pepper to taste

2. Preheat oven to 450 degrees Fahrenheit.

3. Grease or line a baking sheet with parchment paper.

4. Place bread slice in a food processor and allow the motor to run until breadcrumbs form. Transfer to a mixing bowl.

5. Place whole mushrooms in the food processor and pulse until coarsely shredded (to the size of sliced olives). Transfer to a mixing bowl.

6. Repeat with pinto or kidney beans.

7. Combine all ingredients.

8. Using your hands, form patties.

9. Place patties on a cookie sheet, spray with cooking spray, and bake for 10 minutes.

10. Flip, re-spray, and bake for another 8 minutes.

11. Flip, re-spray for the third time and bake 5 minutes more.

BBQ Chop Wrap

- 2 cups chopped romaine lettuce
- 1 small tomato, diced
- ¼ cup canned or cooked black beans
- ¼ cup frozen yellow corn, thawed
- 2 tablespoons BBQ sauce
- 1 whole-wheat wrap or corn tortilla
- ¼ cup crumbled baked corn chips

1. Toss the lettuce, tomatoes, beans, corn, and BBQ sauce together in a mixing bowl, ensuring everything is mostly coated with BBQ sauce.

2. Scoop into a wrap.

3. Add corn chips over the top and roll up.

Salads

Keep Your Heart Beating

- 1 red beet, peeled and shredded
- 1 golden beet, peeled and shredded
- 2 carrots, peeled and shredded
- 2 tablespoons hazelnuts
- 2 tablespoons golden raisins
- ½ teaspoon sea salt

1. In a medium bowl, stir together the red beet, golden beet, carrots, hazelnuts, golden raisins, and salt.

2. Refrigerate for 15 minutes to blend the flavors.

3. Serve.

Mixed Salad

- 1 can (14.5-ounces) whole green beans, drained
- 1 can (16-ounces) kidney beans
- 1 can (14.5-ounces) carrots (or 2 cups steamed fresh carrots)
- 1 cup button mushrooms
- 1 jar (4-ounces) pimiento peppers, drained
- 1 cup water
- ¼ cup coconut oil
- ¼ cup apple cider vinegar
- 2 tablespoons dried oregano
- 1 tablespoon garlic powder
- 1 tablespoon onion powder
- 1 teaspoon sea salt

1. In a medium bowl, combine the green beans, kidney beans, carrots, mushrooms, and pimientos.

2. In a blender, add the water, coconut oil, cider vinegar, oregano, garlic powder, onion powder, and salt.

3. Blend to emulsify the ingredients.

4. Pour the dressing over the vegetables and toss to combine.

5. Cover and chill overnight

Thai Salad

- 4 cups chopped iceberg lettuce
- 1 cup bean sprouts
- 2 carrots, cut into thin slices or spirals
- 1 zucchini, cut into thin strips or spirals
- 1 scallion, finely chopped
- 2 tablespoons almonds, chopped
- Juice of 1 lime
- 1 garlic clove
- 1 teaspoon tamarind paste
- 1 packet stevia
- ½ teaspoon sea salt

1. In a large bowl, combine the lettuce, bean sprouts, carrots, zucchini, scallion, and almonds.

2. In a small food processor bowl, add the lime juice, garlic, tamarind, stevia, and salt. Blend to combine.

3. Pour the dressing over the vegetables and mix thoroughly.

4. Divide evenly between two bowls and serve.

Organic Kale Salad

- Cut kale up as you like it and
- 1 red pepper, diced
- 1 avocado, sliced
- 1 peach, diced
- ½ cup nuts (walnuts or pecans)
- Sweet corn, raw off the cob

Salad dressing:

- 2 tablespoons olive oil (optional)
- 1 tablespoons maple syrup
- 2 tablespoons of apple cider vinegar

* You should massage salad dressing into the mixture with your hands and let it set up in the refrigerator for about 30 minutes.

Healthy Meat Replacements

Kentucky Fried Tofu

- 3 14-ounce packages of firm, extra firm, or super firm tofu, rinsed and drained
- 2-3 teaspoons of soy sauce (or use wheat free tamari or Bragg's liquid amino to keep it gluten free)
- 1 Cup of nutritional yeast for the "breading."

1. Cover a baking tray with parchment paper and preheat the oven to 375 degrees Fahrenheit (temperature may vary depending on the oven).

2. Slice each block of tofu into six rectangular pieces of about half an inch thick.

3. Place soy sauce into a container big enough to accommodate the dipping of tofu slices—an empty tofu carton is what I use, but a plastic food storage container works too.

4. Place nutritional yeast on a large plate.

5. Using wet-hand-dry-hand technique (as pictured above), dip each tofu slice into the soy sauce with one hand and remove to the plate with the yeast (I use my left hand as my wet hand).

6. Using the other (right) hand, cover the tofu with the yeast "breading," ensuring that each slice is well coated.

7. Place "breaded" tofu slices on the baking tray lined with parchment paper, ensuring that none of the pieces touch.

8. Bake in the oven for 30–60 minutes until the yeast sticks to the tofu and not the paper, creating a thin layer of crust around each slice.

9. If the yeast sticks to the parchment paper, continue to bake until yeast clings to the tofu.

10. Once yeast sticks to the tofu, gently flip each slice.

11. Bake for another 30–45 minutes until tofu is adequately dehydrated and yeast sticks to the tofu and not the parchment paper.

12. Tofu can be enjoyed as "steaks" or cut into cubes once it cools a little.

13. Total cook time will depend on the oven and type of tofu used. Super-firm tofu requires about an hour of total cook time, while firm or extra-firm tofu requires about 1 hour and 45 minutes of total cook time to adequately dehydrate.

Seitan . . . What Is It?

Seitan is food with a long history. Although not widely known in the West, seitan has been traditional fare in China, Korea, Japan, Middle Eastern countries, and most other places where wheat is a staple product. In North America, the Mormons and the Seventh-day Adventists eat seitan frequently. Seitan—gluten that has been extracted from wheat flour and then cooked—comes to the United States from Japan, where once it would have been prepared by vegetarian Buddhist monks. It is also known simply as gluten or "wheat meat." However, we prefer to use the Japanese name, even though technically the word seitan refers to gluten that has been cooked in soy sauce.

If you want great seitan, you have to make it.

The Basic Ingredients

Seitan is vital wheat gluten and water. Many seitan recipes include some chickpea or garbanzo flour, which is used to give the seitan a lighter texture. This can also be done by adding nutritional yeast with the added benefit of lots of vitamins. The most common wet ingredients used in seitan are water, vegetable broth, olive oil and tamari, soy sauce, or liquid aminos. Together, these dry and wet ingredients will be combined to make the seitan dough. Seitan that is chewier, such as is used to create "ribs," requires less liquid than the soft, tender seitan you would want for a stew.

Season Inside and Out

One of the advantages of making your seitan is that you can season it on the inside as well as the outside. If I want my seitan to have a "beefy" flavor, I add tomato paste to the dough. Sometimes I also add vegan Worcestershire sauce for that deep umami flavor. Then I choose herbs and spices associated with beef such as cumin, coriander, oregano, and paprika. Vegan "beefy" broth can also be used instead of vegetable broth to intensify the flavor. On the other hand, if I want my seitan to be more like chicken, pork or just more neutral, I will use vegan "chicken" flavored broth and herbs such as thyme and sage.

After the seitan is made, it gets more seasoning depending on how I am going to prepare it. You do not want to eat seitan without cooking it somehow. At the very least, sauté the seitan in some oil to give it a nice crust and added flavor. Chunks of seitan for a stew will get browned in seasoned flour before adding any liquids. Sliced seitan gets seasoned with garlic powder, celery salt, black pepper, and cayenne when I am making a French dip sandwich. Seitan ribs and steaks are flavored with spice rubs and/or marinades. Food is all about texture and flavor, so be generous when it comes to seasoning your seitan.

You Need to Knead

Seitan is a dough, and like most dough, it needs to be kneaded. Kneading helps develop the gluten and brings elasticity and stretch into the dough. The longer you knead the dough, the more gluten you develop, leading to a chewier seitan. If you want a less chewy and more tender seitan, knead it for a shorter period. Most recipes require kneading the dough for an average of 3 minutes, followed by a 10-minute rest period and then a bit more kneading. As you knead the seitan, you will feel it change from a wet, sticky mixture to firmer dough; that is the gluten developing. You will be able to stretch the dough and watch it snap back into place; that is the elasticity.

After kneading my seitan, I place it in my Instant Pot with 4 cups of broth and spices to flavor it from the outside. Turn the Instant Pot on manual, select 20 minutes, and wait for it to complete. After Instant Pot is finished, I let it cool. You can eat it right away, but it is better the next day.

Vegan Pork Anyone?

The technique for mixing this dough creates a stringy texture that is the perfect answer for pulled pork, potstickers, and dumplings. You can eat it as is or shred it, grind it, or marinate it. The liquid from cooking results in a rich broth full of depth and flavor, making it a perfect base for soups.

- 1 cup water
- ⅓ cup oil
- 2 tablespoons organic sugar or stevia
- 1 tablespoon soy sauce
- 1 teaspoon liquid smoke
- 2 teaspoons onion powder
- 2 teaspoons sea salt
- 2 ¼ cups vital wheat gluten
- Oil, for cooking

1. Mix the water, oil, stevia, soy sauce, liquid smoke, onion powder, and 1 teaspoon of the salt in a large bowl.

2. Add about 2 cups of the vital wheat gluten and mix well.

3. Finally, add the remaining quarter cup of gluten, working it in with your hands, breaking and stretching it until no dry flour shows. The dough will be rough and stringy (it is all in the mixing technique, so don't dump all the gluten in there at once!).

4. Heat a deep skillet over medium heat with a little oil and cook the seitan pieces on both sides until browned.

5. Cover with water, add the remaining 1 teaspoon salt, put a lid on the pan, and simmer for 30 minutes to 1 hour, until cooked through. You can check by cutting a piece in half; there should be tiny air pockets throughout.

Seitan Ribs Aplenty

- ¼ cup soy sauce
- 3 tablespoons nutritional yeast
- 2 tablespoons smooth peanut butter
- 2 tablespoons tomato paste
- 1 tablespoon white, chickpea, or red miso

- 4 or 5 garlic cloves
- 1 ¼ cups water
- 2 ½ to 3 cups vital wheat gluten
- Oil, for cooking (optional)

Sauce

- 3 ½ to 4 cups barbecue sauce or your favorite store-bought variety
- 2 cups water

1. In a food processor or blender, combine the soy sauce, nutritional yeast, peanut butter, tomato paste, miso, garlic, and water and process until a smooth and creamy slurry is created.

2. If you are using a food processor, just keep everything in there; if using a blender, pour it out into a large mixing bowl.

3. Add 2 and a half cups of the gluten to the slurry and mix well, either using the food processor or by hand in the bowl.

4. If you are using a food processor, keep pulsing to knead the dough, adding a little more gluten flour as necessary to form a stiff dough (the more gluten you add, the chewier your ribs will be, so you can control how tender or chewy you want them). It may form one ball in the center or break up into little beads; if it breaks up, all you have to do is push it together with your hands. If you are mixing it by hand, knead it in the bowl for several minutes until it becomes smooth.

5. Preheat oven to 350 degrees Fahrenheit.

6. Lightly grease an 8-inch by 8-inch baking dish and set aside.

7. Transfer mixture into the greased baking dish and flatten so that it is spread evenly across the entire dish.

8. Use a knife to make one lengthwise cut across the dough, then cut evenly crosswise to make 1-inch slices. (You do not need to pull them apart; you just want the ability to easily separate them after grilling.)

9. Place dish in the preheated oven and bake for 25 minutes.

10. While the ribs are baking, heat up your grill or lightly oil a grill pan.

11. Remove ribs from oven and brush the tops with barbecue sauce.

12. Place ribs sauce-side down on heated grill (or a grill pan on the stove over medium heat), and brush the tops with more barbecue sauce.

13. When the bottom of the ribs are deeply browned (about 5–6 minutes), flip over and cook the other side until brown.

14. Remove from heat and serve immediately, with more barbecue sauce if desired.

Sweet Treats

Banana-Coconut Crème Pie

Crust:

- 1 ½ cups macadamia nuts
- ½ cup shredded coconut
- ½ teaspoon salt
- 3 tablespoons maple syrup
- 1 tablespoon coconut oil, melted
- 1 teaspoon vanilla extract

Banana Crème Filling:

- 3 cups soaked cashews
- 2 cups mashed banana
- 1 cup maple syrup
- 2 teaspoons vanilla extract

- 1 tablespoon lemon juice
- ¼ teaspoon salt
- ½ cup coconut oil, melted

Coconut Crème Filling:

- 1 ½ cups soaked cashews
- 1 ½ cups coconut milk
- ½ cup maple syrup
- 1 tablespoon vanilla extract

- 1 teaspoon lemon juice
- 1 cup coconut oil, melted
- Pinch of salt
- 1 banana, sliced for layering

1. To make the crust: In a food processor, blend the macadamia nuts, shredded coconut, and salt until they become crumbly flour. Add the maple syrup, coconut oil, and vanilla; lightly pulse until all ingredients are well mixed but only stick together when pressed between your fingers.

2. To make the banana crème filling: Blend all the ingredients except the coconut oil in a mixer until smooth. Add the coconut oil and blend until combined. Put in the refrigerator for a few minutes to set.

3. To make the coconut crème: Blend the first five ingredients in a mixer until smooth. Then add coconut oil and salt and continue to blend until completely combined. Put in the refrigerator for a few minutes to set.

4. To assemble: Press crust into a 9-inch tart pan with a removable bottom. Pour in banana crème filling. Top with banana slices. Top with coconut crème. Let set in the refrigerator for at least 30 minutes before serving.

Stone Fruit Pie

Crust:

- 2 ¼ cups almonds, soaked overnight and dehydrated
- 3 tablespoons maple syrup
- 1 tablespoon coconut oil, melted
- ¼ teaspoon salt

Filling:

- 3 cups cashews, soaked 1 to 2 hours
- ½ cup lemon juice
- ¾ cup agave nectar, maple syrup, or honey
- 1 tablespoon vanilla extract
- 1 teaspoon salt
- 1 vanilla bean, scraped
- 1 teaspoon cinnamon
- ¼ teaspoon nutmeg
- ¾ cup coconut oil, melted

Topping:

- 2 cups sliced mixed stone fruit, such as plums, apricots, peaches, or cherries
- ¼ cup agave nectar, maple syrup, or honey
- 1 tablespoon lemon juice

1. To make the crust: Place prepared almonds in a food processor and pulse into a coarse flour. Add the remaining ingredients and lightly pulse until well mixed. Press into a 9-inch tart pan with a removable bottom.

2. To make the filling: Blend all ingredients except coconut oil in a mixer until smooth. Then add the coconut oil and blend until completely combined, but do not over blend.

3. To make the fruit topping: Toss sliced fruit with maple syrup and lemon juice. Pour filling into crust, then arrange sliced fruit on top.

Triple-Layer Cacao Cake

Wet ingredients:

- 3 cups date paste
- ½ cup almond milk
- ½ cup maple syrup
- 5 tablespoons vanilla extract
- ½ cup coconut oil, melted

Dry Ingredients:

- 4 cups almond flour
- 4 cups hazelnut flour
- 1 cup coconut powder
- 1 cup cacao powder
- 1 teaspoon salt
- ¼ cup Irish Moss paste can be used with wet ingredients or ¼ cup flax meal with the dry. This is optional and creates a fluffier mixture.

Fudge Frosting:

- 2 cups cashew flour
- 2 cups almond milk
- ½ cup maple syrup
- 4 tablespoons vanilla extract
- 1 cup cacao powder
- ¼ teaspoon salt
- ¾ cup coconut oil, melted chocolate maple glaze

1. **Preparing Wet Ingredients:** In a mixer, thoroughly blend all the wet ingredients except for the coconut oil until smooth. Then add the coconut oil and continue to blend until well combined.

2. **Cake Batter:** In a mixer or food processor, mix the dry ingredients until thoroughly combined. Slowly add the wet ingredients. It is better to use a standing mixer as this will keep the mixture lighter and more fluffy, but if you do not have a standing mixer, the batter can be made in a food processor if you lightly pulse the wet ingredients in. You do not want a dense, heavily blended mixture.

3. **Frosting:** In a mixer, thoroughly blend all the ingredients except for the coconut oil and chocolate maple glaze until smooth. Then add the coconut oil and continue to blend until well combined and creamy.

Place in the refrigerator for 30 – 60 minutes until slightly firm but still spreadable.

4. **Assembly:** Divide cake batter into fourths. Press one layer of batter in a 9-inch springform pan and alternate with frosting. Refrigerate until just before serving and glaze with chocolate maple glaze.

German Chocolate Cake

Wet Ingredients:

- 3 cups date paste
- ½ cup almond milk
- ½ cup maple syrup
- 5 tablespoons vanilla extract
- ½ cup coconut oil, melted

Dry Ingredients:

- 7 cups almond flour
- 2 cups shredded coconut (powdered in a mixer)
- 1 cup cacao powder
- 1 teaspoon salt
- ¼ cup Irish Moss paste can be used with wet ingredients or ¼ cup flax meal with the dry. This is optional and creates a fluffier mixture.

Pecan Coconut Frosting:

- 2 cups cashew flour
- 1 ½ cups pecan milk
- 1 cup maple syrup
- 4 tablespoons vanilla extract
- Pinch salt
- ¾ cup coconut oil, melted
- 1 cup chopped pecans
- 2 cups shredded coconut
- 1 cup caramel (optional)

1. **Preparing Wet Ingredients:** In a mixer, thoroughly blend all the wet ingredients, except the coconut oil, until smooth. Then add the coconut oil and continue to blend until well combined.

2. **Cake Batter:** In a mixer or food processor, mix the dry ingredients until thoroughly combined. Slowly add the wet ingredients. It is better

to use a standing mixer as this will keep the mixture lighter and more fluffy, but if you do not have a standing mixer, the batter can be made in a food processor if you lightly pulse the wet ingredients in. You do not want a dense, heavily blended mixture.

3. **Frosting:** In a mixer, thoroughly blend the first five ingredients until smooth. Then add the coconut oil and continue to blend until well combined and creamy. Stir in chopped pecans and shredded coconut. Place in the refrigerator for 30 – 60 minutes until slightly firm, but still spreadable.

4. **Assembly:** Divide cake batter into thirds. Press one layer of batter in a 9-inch springform pan and alternate with frosting until you have made three layers. Refrigerate until just before serving. To make the cake extra decadent, serve with caramel.

Candied Carrot-Ginger Cake

Wet Ingredients:

- 3 cups date paste
- ¼ cup ginger juice
- ½ cup apple juice
- 2 tablespoons vanilla extract
- ½ cup coconut oil, melted Dry Ingredients
- 7 cups almond flour
- 1 cup pecans, soaked and dehydrated
- 1 cup walnuts, soaked and dehydrated
- 2 ½ cups shredded carrots
- ¾ cup raisins, chopped
- 1 ½ tablespoons cinnamon
- 1 tablespoon grated ginger
- 1 teaspoon nutmeg
- 1 teaspoon cloves
- 1 teaspoon salt
- ¼ cup Irish Moss paste can be used with wet ingredients or ¼ cup flax meal with the dry. This is optional and creates a fluffier mixture.

Ginger Cream Frosting:

- 1 ½ cups cashew flour
- ½ cup macadamia nuts
- 1 cup almond milk
- 1 cup maple syrup
- 3 tablespoons ginger juice
- 1 tablespoon grated ginger
- ¼ cup lemon juice
- 1 tablespoon vanilla extract
- ¼ teaspoon salt
- 1 cup coconut oil, melted

1. **Preparing Wet Ingredients:** In a mixer, thoroughly blend all the wet ingredients, except for the coconut oil, until smooth. Then add the coconut oil and continue to blend until well combined.

2. **Cake Batter:** In a mixer or food processor, mix the almond flour, pecans, and walnuts until thoroughly combined. You want the walnuts and pecans to still be slightly chunky. Mix the carrots, raisins, and spices in the mixing bowl of a standing mixer. You do not want to over process these ingredients. Slowly add the wet ingredients. Do not make this cake in a food processor. If you do not have a standing mixer, this recipe is best mixed by hand so that it remains fluffy and crumbly.

3. **Frosting:** In a mixer, thoroughly blend all the wet ingredients, except for the coconut oil, until smooth. Then add the coconut oil and continue to blend until well combined and creamy. Place in the refrigerator for 30 – 60 minutes until slightly firm, but still spreadable.

4. **Assembly:** Divide cake batter in half. Press one layer of batter in a 9-inch springform pan and alternate with one-third of the frosting. Add second cake layer. Refrigerate until just before serving, remove from springform pan, and frost with remaining frosting.

We are living in a very exciting time with so much to eat and so many great recipes; I could not cover nearly as many as I wanted to because they are just too many. So, a big super size thank you to everyone that provided their favorite recipe for my book. To see more recipes go to my website: www.jamesjazzyjordan.com.

About the Author

James "Jazzy" Jordan

Veganism is my way of life, and I have tried almost everything a plant-based diet has to offer. In 1990, I started out as a vegetarian with little knowledge about the lifestyle. At that time, there were not very many vegetarian restaurants and no vegan or raw food restaurants at all, so it was a journey. But, when I decide to do something, I stay with it. Sometimes when I was traveling and there was nothing super healthy to eat, I would go to Burger King and get a Whopper® without the meat patty to have something to keep me going.

I have traveled the world to learn about a plant-base lifestyle and the benefits. I have owned every gadget: juicers, blenders, dehydrators, food processors . . . you name it, I have it, so I can tell you which is best and the ones to leave in the store.

I am a John Maxwell certified coach, a teacher, speaker, and bestselling author. I offer workshops, seminars, keynotes, and coaching to aid your personal and professional growth. As a passionate entrepreneur and business consultant, I equip my clients with the tools necessary to achieve their desired results.

I am no stranger to creating success. From marketing, promotions, radio broadcasting, and retail, to record executive, songwriter, composer and record producer, I was listed as one of the "Bosses of The Decade" by Jet magazine along with the likes of Berry Gordy, Cathy Hughes, Bob Johnson, Quincy Jones and others. This list of trailblazing entertainment power players has made history and billions of dollars in the entertainment industry. Personally, I have amassed over 2 billion dollars in record sales cumulatively over the course of my career. Maximizing the operating performance of organizations and helping them to achieve their financial goals is my strong suit.

I was also honored as "An American Icon" by Rep. Shelia Jackson-Lee at the U.S. House of Representatives for my service to the music industry. In other ventures, I am one of only two African Americans to have ownership of a car entrant into the prestigious Indianapolis 500 race.

I went from working in a record store to being the program and music director and afternoon announcer in my hometown radio station, to Executive Vice President at Jive and Verity Records. Taking it all the way to the upper echelons of the music, film, and entertainment industries, my distinguished career spans over 30 years. I am an entertainment business professional who has collaborated with many of America's top entertainers. I have worked with Will Smith, R. Kelly, Marvin Sapp, John P. Kee, Joe, Will Downing, Salt n Pepa, Kirk Franklin, Yolanda Adams, Fred Hammond, and Donnie McClurkin to name a few. I have collected more gold and platinum records than can be displayed on walls of my home.

Frequently Asked Questions

1. Where do we get iron, if not from red meat?

The most substantial sources of iron are "greens and beans," that is green leafy vegetables and anything from the bean group. These foods also bring us calcium and other important minerals. Vegetables, beans, and other foods provide all the iron you need. In fact, studies show that vegetarians and vegans tend to get more iron than meat eaters. Vitamin C increases iron absorption. Meanwhile, dairy products reduce iron absorption significantly. There are two forms of iron: plants have non-heme iron, which is more absorbable when the body is low in iron and less absorbable when the body already has enough iron. This allows the body to regulate its iron balance. On the other hand, meats have heme iron, which barges right into your bloodstream whether you need it or not. The problem is that many people have too much iron stored in their bodies. Excess iron can spark the production of free radicals that accelerate aging, increase the risk of heart disease, and cause other problems. So, while iron is important to avoid anemia, you also do not want to be iron overloaded. It is probably best to have your hemoglobin on the low end of the normal range. If your energy is good and your hemoglobin and hematocrit are at the low end of normal, that is likely the best place to be.

2. What is the best source of calcium?

The same green leafy vegetables and legumes that provide iron are also good sources of calcium, for the most part, and absorption is typically better from these sources than from dairy products. Broccoli, Brussels sprouts, kale, and other common greens have highly absorbable calcium.

To aid calcium absorption:

- Eliminate animal protein. For a variety of reasons, animal protein causes calcium loss.
- Limit salt intake. Sodium tends to cause the body to lose calcium in the urine.
- Eat plenty of fruits and vegetables. People who eat lots of vegetables and fruits are less likely to have bone breaks. Part of the reason may be that vegetables and fruit contain vitamin C, which is essential for building collagen, the underlying bone matrix.
- Do not smoke. Studies have shown that women who smoke one pack of cigarettes a day have 5 to 10 percent less bone density at menopause than nonsmokers.

3. Is it healthy for a pregnant or nursing mother to eat a plant-based diet? How about kids?

According to the American Dietetic Association position paper on vegetarian and vegan diets:

"Well-planned vegan and other types of vegetarian diets are appropriate for all stages of the life-cycle including during pregnancy, lactation, infancy, childhood, and adolescence. Vegetarian diets offer some nutritional benefits, including lower levels of saturated fat, cholesterol, and animal protein as well as higher levels of carbohydrates, fiber, magnesium, potassium, folate, antioxidants such as vitamins C and E, and phytochemicals.[11]"

---

11 Position of the American Dietetic Association and ... (n.d.). Retrieved from https://www.ncbi.nlm.nih.gov/pubmed/12778049/

"Vegetarians have been reported to have lower body mass indices than non-vegetarians, as well as lower rates of death from ischemic heart disease, lower blood cholesterol levels, lower blood pressure, and lower rates of hypertension, type 2 diabetes, and prostate and colon cancer.[12]"

In the seventh edition of Dr. Benjamin Spock's *Baby and Child Care*—the last edition published during Dr. Spock's lifetime—he spelled out some good advice: he recommended that children be served plant-based diets.

4. Do I need to take any particular vitamins or minerals because of eating this way?

Vegans generally have better overall vitamin intake, compared with meat eaters. Meat has essentially no vitamin C and is low in many other vitamins as well. In contrast, vegetables, fruits, and legumes (beans, peas, and lentils) are vitamin-rich. In controlled studies, people switching to vegan diets typically increase their intake of several vitamins and reduce their intake of the undesirables—saturated fat and cholesterol, in particular.

Even so, two vitamins deserve special comment: Vitamin B12 is made, not by plants or animals, but by bacteria. Animal products contain B12 made by the bacteria in their intestinal tracts. A more healthy source is any common multiple vitamin. B12 supplements are also widely available. Vitamin D normally comes from exposure to the sun. About fifteen minutes of direct sunlight on your face and arms each day gives you all the vitamin D you need. However, if you are indoors much of the day or live in an area where sunlight is limited, it is important to take a supplement.

5. How much protein do I need and where is the best place to get it?

A plant-based diet easily provides all the protein the body needs. There is no need for meat, dairy products, or eggs for protein, and you are better

---

12 Position of the American Dietetic Association and ... (n.d.). Retrieved from https://www.ncbi.nlm.nih.gov/pubmed/12778049/

off without them. Vegetables, grains, and beans give you plenty of protein, even if you are active and athletic. The normal mixtures of food people choose from day to day easily satisfy protein needs. Protein is made up of amino acids. Each amino acid molecule is like a bead, and many amino acids together make up the protein chain. There are many different amino acids, and all of the essential ones are found in plants. The bottom line is to have a healthy mix of vegetables, beans, whole grains, and fruits, and protein takes care of itself.

6. WHAT'S THE DEAL WITH SOY?

Soy products have been around for thousands of years and are a dietary staple in many regions of Asia. Research has shown that people in these regions have lower rates of heart disease, breast and prostate cancer, fewer hip fractures and fewer hot flashes. Also, dozens of clinical studies have indicated the health benefits of diets rich in soy. Some have raised the question as to whether soy has untoward effects. Happily, these concerns have been set aside. Girls who consume soy products in adolescence have about a 30 percent reduction in breast cancer risk as adults. Women previously diagnosed with breast cancer have a significantly greater survival if they include soy in their diets, compared with women who tend not to use soy products. However, if a person is uncertain or simply does not want to include soy, I always remind them that a vegan diet does not mean joining the Soy Promotion Society.

7. SOMETIMES EATING LOTS OF VEGETABLES, BEANS, OR SOY PRODUCTS GIVES ME UNCOMFORTABLE GAS; HOW DO YOU AVOID THIS?

The problem with gassiness can often be found with beans. They should not be excluded from the diet, however, because they are great sources of protein, calcium, and iron, among other nutrients. However, if you are new to beans, it is good to have them in small portions and always very well cooked. A well-cooked bean is very soft, with no hint of crunchiness. As time goes on, your digestive tract adjusts, so a bean that may cause a problem today may be better tolerated later on. Also, cruciferous vegetables can cause indigestion for some people. The answer is simply to cook them well. This group includes broccoli, cauliflower, Brussels sprouts, kale, and cabbage, among others. It is common for people to eat them raw or only slightly cooked, but they can easily cause gassiness or bloating. Cook them well, and the problem usually disappears. Later on, you can experiment again with less-cooked vegetables. On the good side, brown rice is very easily digested, and a great food to prioritize. Brown rice is best. Also, cooked green, yellow, and orange vegetables are very easily digested. Fruits vary. Some people do very well with raw fruit; others have more difficulty at first. If you are new to any particular fruit, you might have smaller servings at first, then gradually increase.

Take your health seriously, if you take care of your health your health will take care of you. Health is wealth.

For Information go to my website: www.jamesjazzyjordan.com for recipes, food demos, and contact information.

ACKNOWLEDGMENTS

I owe a debt of gratitude to so many, so let's start at the beginning. Professor Linda Beasley, Thank you for introducing me to the plant-base lifestyle 27 years ago. Special thanks to my niece, Meagan Jordan, for her help with my book; she was invaluable. I also want to thank Jessica Moses and Barbara Inchcliff for their support. To all the great leaders in the field of veganism, I simply say thank you for all that you do. A huge thanks to everyone that contribute to this book, by submitting recipes, ideas, love and support. To my family, I could never do anything without you guys. My children James, Laura, Alison and the grandchildren, I love you all, you are the wind beneath my wings.

I also want to thank Rob, David, and Randy of Best Seller Publishing for their wonderful work—you guys are the best.

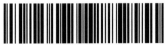
Made in the USA
San Bernardino, CA
23 March 2017